The Natural Baby

Nov 17

For Ella, Yasmin, Max
and Jasmine

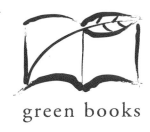

green books

The Natural Baby

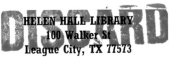
A gentle guide
to conception,
pregnancy, birth
and beyond

Samantha Quinn
and Holly Daffurn

Green Books
An imprint of UIT Cambridge Ltd
www.greenbooks.co.uk

PO Box 145, Cambridge CB4 1GQ, England
+44 (0) 1223 302 041

First published in 2017, in England.

Samantha Quinn and Holly Daffurn have asserted their moral rights under the Copyright, Designs and Patents Act 1988.

All of the photographs in this book, (apart from the photo on page 11 taken from Shutterstock) were taken by Holly Daffurn and she retains all the rights to the photos.

Design by Mad-i-Creative
www.mad-i-creative.co.uk

ISBN: 978 0 85784 401 9 (paperback)
ISBN: 978 0 85784 402 6 (ePub)
ISBN: 978 0 85784 403 3 (PDF)
Also available for Kindle.

Disclaimer: the advice herein is believed to be correct at the time of printing, but the authors and publisher accept no liability for actions inspired by this book.

10 9 8 7 6 5 4 3 2 1

Foreword

Everything changes when we become a parent; we become responsible for a tiny dependent being. It's a parental instinct to want to create the healthiest, safest place for this little person to grow up in, and many of us turn to a greener lifestyle to ensure our child's wellbeing.

There is no one way to raise a child naturally but there are some common practices such as extended breastfeeding, babywearing, co-sleeping, using alternative medicine, choosing reusable nappies or elimination communication, spending as much time outside as possible, going screen free and growing or buying organic produce.

Inside this book Samantha Quinn and Holly Daffurn empower parents with the information and wisdom to help them make the best choices for their families. As a duo Samantha and Holly have the perfect set of complementary skills and knowledge to write about natural parenting. And with four children between them they share great passion for this way of life too. I love the gentle affirmative style of writing; here is a book that will act like a best friend. Imagine being taken by the hand and gently guided along the right parenting path.

One of the best aspects of the book that you hold in your hands is the space given to self-care. The surest way that we can create a happy, healthy home for our new child is to care for ourselves; to ensure that we are getting our own physical and emotional needs met. The most important thing to learn as a parent is to Think Oxygen; during safety announcements we are encouraged to secure our own source of oxygen before administering our children's. We cannot care for another if we are depleted ourselves. Here you'll be given the practical tools and techniques to ensure that you are looking after yourself from day one.

Anxious about what you should eat for optimum health during pregnancy? The chapters on pregnancy are packed with well-researched and practical information. Want to know how to have the most natural labour? Find the active birthing positions and recommendations in the chapter on Birth. Concerned about what to feed your baby who's starting to show an interest in food? Follow the simple step-by-step weaning process here and try out some of the nourishing first food ideas. Throughout this book new dads will find the Natural Dad sections reassuring, along with the photographs of real-life fathers! This whole package is warm and welcoming, inviting and inspiring and designed to make you feel better.

And this book is just the start of a great collaboration; be sure to visit the website, join the social media channels and look out for a whole series of books. I am excited to see what these two passionate women have planned next.

Melissa Corkhill

Editor of The Green Parent magazine
www.thegreenparent.co.uk

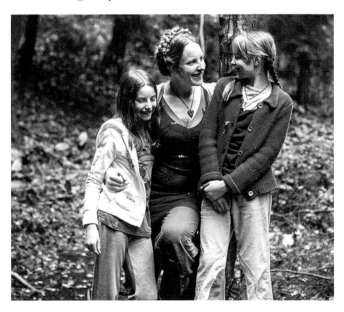

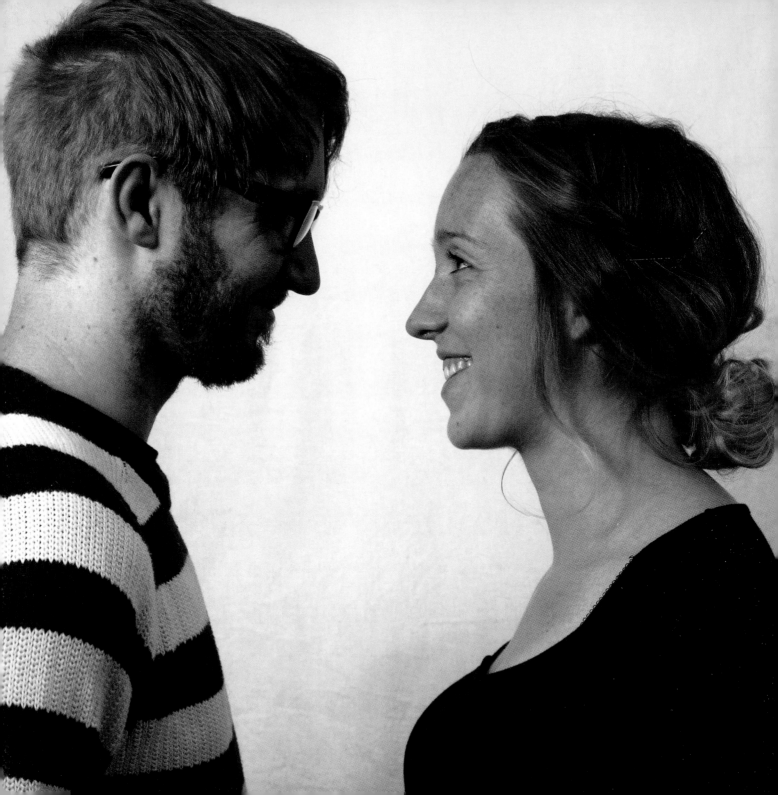

Contents

Introduction

When it comes to parenting, the combination of choices and responsibility can feel overwhelming. The key is to do what feels right for you and your baby. Natural babycare choices combined with gentle parenting will help your child to grow up well rounded and happy.

Natural parenting is about making conscious decisions on your parenting journey. The focus is on environmentally responsible choices, healthy eating, holistic practices and striving to find balance. It is about keeping your mind as healthy as your body, and making informed decisions that help you to keep your children as healthy and happy as possible, while strengthening the bonding process between you.

We will guide you through the entire journey from when you first decide to have a baby to life with your newborn. You may decide to follow every last piece of advice that we give you; you may prefer to pick the parts that fit in with your lifestyle. We start before conception, take you through the pregnancy, through an active birth (where you are encouraged to move about freely during labour and to follow your natural instincts) and into the postnatal period as you settle in with your baby. We combine personal stories, medical research and physiological facts such as your baby's week-by-week development and the science behind breastfeeding. We look at the emotional and practical side of parenting, and address natural ways to relieve the less welcome parts of pregnancy such as heartburn and morning sickness.

Each chapter takes you one step further along your parenting journey, with plenty of advice on what to expect, how to feel your best and what you'll need to consider. Few books address the role of the father in natural parenting so we have included a special section to give dads advice and support along the way.

You should only use essential oils in pregnancy if you have no health concerns or complications. If you are at all unsure you should always consult your doctor.

This book is the labour of love of two passionate and devoted natural parenting aficionados who are also blessed to be mums. Before we begin, these are our stories:

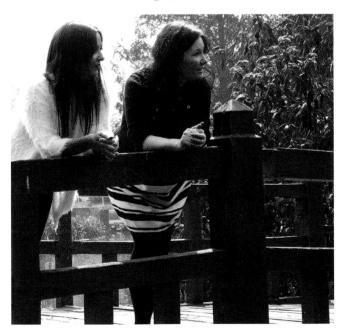

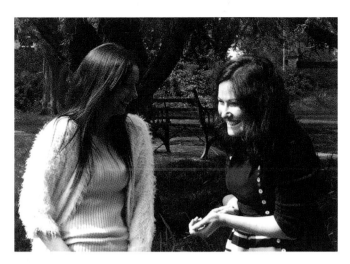

Sam

Having Ella was one of the most amazing moments of my life. I was a little apprehensive about birth. After all, movie births always seem so dramatic, waters breaking in the supermarket, deliveries on the bathroom floor, partners who pass out. But even though Ella was born early, her birth went as smoothly as it could have done for a premature baby.

After Ella was born she was transferred to the special-care baby unit. Although it was hard not being able to cuddle my child when I wanted to, the nurse caring for Ella introduced me to baby massage. She taught me about the power of touch and how it can really help to stabilize a baby's breathing and heart rate, and encourage their physical and emotional development. Massage helped to calm Ella and made what precious time we had together more enjoyable.

When I brought Ella home, I remembered what the nurse had told me about natural babycare. Strapping Ella into her sling I headed off to the local library to research holistic parenting. A whole new world opened up and from there I created my own natural colic relief massage and learned how to blend organic baby oils and balms to help her sensitive skin. As Ella thrived I went back to college to learn more about natural therapies, and eventually I became a holistic therapist specializing in pregnancy and postnatal care in west Sussex, UK.

When I became pregnant with my second child, Yasmin, I was able to put everything I had learned into practice. I blended juices for the added nutrients that we needed, I became stronger through good nutrition and yoga, and I practised herbalism (the medicinal and therapeutic use of plants to treat common health issues). To offset the challenges of pregnancy, I used both aromatherapy and hypnobirthing so that my mind was as prepared as my body. This time round I was enjoying a truly holistic approach to childbirth.

After my third child, Max came along I decided to take my passion to the next level. This was the trigger for Mumma Love Organics, a skincare product range to help parents heal their babies' common ailments naturally. So far we have won a number of awards including gold in the UK's Mother&Baby Awards for best baby skincare brand. All products come with a directional baby massage guide to enhance their effectiveness (for more information visit www.mummaloveorganics.com).

I love the fact that it was my children who introduced me to the rich new world of holistic therapies that I couldn't now be without.

Holly

I think the term holistic parenting can conjure up a vision of an impossibly healthy couple who are more focused on their lifestyle choices than their kids. In fact, a holistic approach has the potential to cure the symptoms of a health problem and its cause (unlike much conventional medicine). The holistic view takes into account everything from diet to emotions, from stress to lifestyle; it treats the whole person, not just the symptoms, so ensures that nothing is missed. For me, holistic parenting is about raising your children with equal consideration for their physical, emotional and mental well-being. It is about making the best choices that you can without getting hung up on what you can't manage. So don't aim for perfection, it doesn't exist.

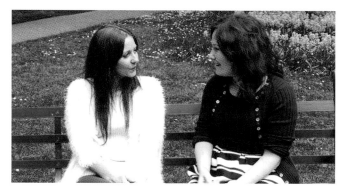

With social media forming such an integral part of our culture, everyone seems intent on projecting their best side nowadays. Many women feel overwhelmed with motherhood simply because everyone else appears to make it look so easy. Sam and I haven't written this book because we are flawless parents, but because we found natural methods and complementary therapies to be so very beneficial when pregnant and raising our own children.

I'd like to let you in on a couple of home truths. I humbly admit that I contributed to the vast number of nappies in landfill. When my daughter was born we were living in a tiny flat with little space to dry reusables. Instead of washing nappies I spent more time breastfeeding, puréeing vegetables and interacting with Jasmine. Later, I stopped breastfeeding at four months when the mastitis got the better of me. It was a beautiful start, but I'm glad I knew when it was the right time to stop breastfeeding. I don't regret the choices I made.

I was raised in a house where lavender oil was used to treat headaches, arnica cream was used for burns, and ear infections were treated with belladonna. By the time I had reached high school my mum's yoga books had migrated to my room.

Aromatherapy helped me through exam stress, Bach Flower Remedies were administered before my driving test, and a glossy book on kundalini yoga was one of my first purchases with my student loan.

When I became pregnant at 19, I learned all about natural birthing techniques and followed my instincts to guide me through an uncomplicated labour. After my daughter was old enough to attend nursery, I studied complementary therapies and nutrition.

Having run my own mobile massage practice, I went on to teach classes for pregnant women in children's centres, covering yoga, breathing exercises, relaxation and birthing techniques. Finally, I was able to share my passion.

There is no such person as the perfect parent and striving for unreachable ideals will ultimately just make you feel exhausted and inadequate. We're not here to tell you what to do but to share the knowledge that we have picked up along the way. No matter where you are on your parenting and natural health journey, we hope you find this book valuable.

A note about measurements we use:

A standard glass is 250ml (8fl oz).
A standard tablespoon is 15ml (½fl oz).

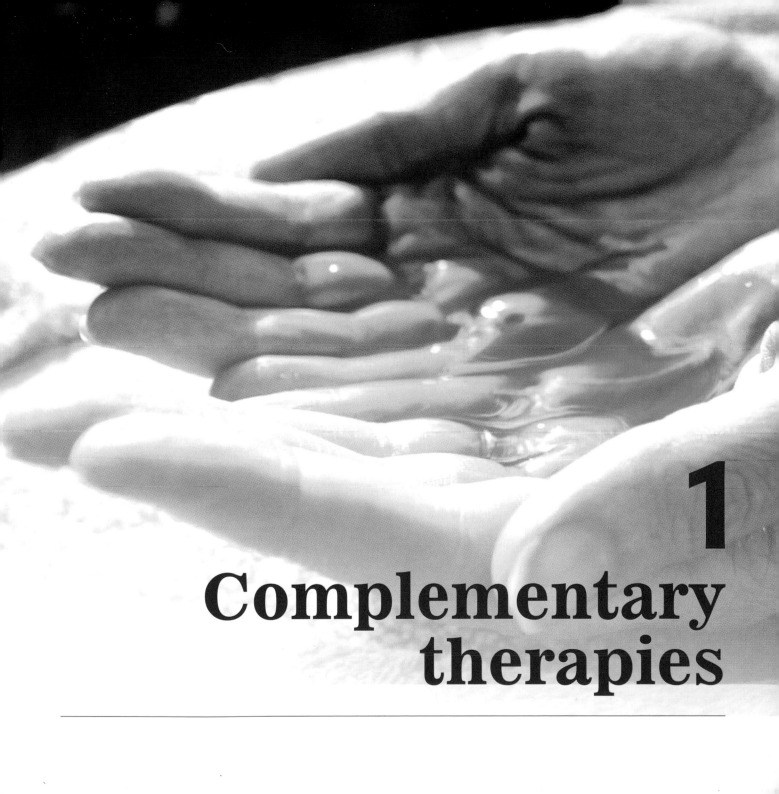

1
Complementary therapies

1
Complementary therapies

Complementary therapies – treatments used alongside conventional medicine – have been used for centuries, some studies suggest as far back as 10,000 BC, in civilizations including China, Egypt, Japan and Native America.

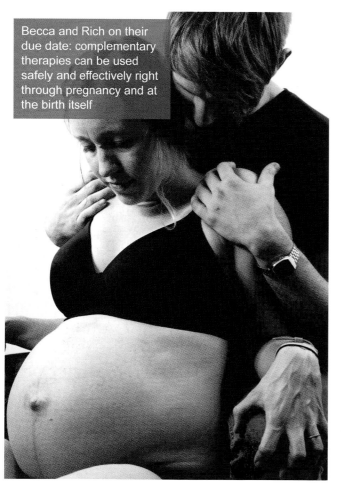

Becca and Rich on their due date: complementary therapies can be used safely and effectively right through pregnancy and at the birth itself

These alternative therapies are still viewed by some doctors with a degree of cynicism but they are often very effective. For example, massage therapy has been found to decrease pain, depression and anxiety in pregnancy. Research also shows that during labour, massage therapy can result in significantly less pain, less need for medication and labours that are on average three hours shorter.[1] So many medicines tend to be off-limits when you're pregnant as they may harm your unborn child. Complementary therapies are gentle and non-intrusive and can make you feel more in tune with your body.

Thanks to improvements in medicine, sanitation, nutrition and technology, giving birth in the twenty-first century is safer in most countries than ever before. And yet, however fantastic as these medical advances are, sometimes clinical procedures can take over what the body is usually capable of doing itself. The UK's National Institute for Health and Care Excellence (NICE) conclude that for low-risk women, birth is generally very safe for both mother and baby, and mothers should be free to choose a home birth and be supported in their choice.[2] The *Journal of Midwifery & Women's Health* in the US confirms that among low-risk women, planned home births result in low rates of interventions without an increase in adverse outcomes for mothers and babies.[3] In 2012 in the USA[4] and Canada,[5] less than 2 per cent of births were out-of-hospital. In Australia around 1,000 women each year choose a home birth.[6] In

2010 the national home birth rate in New Zealand was 3.2 per cent of women.[7]

Although it is now common to write your own birth plan, labour can be an unpredictable experience and more and more women are also proactive leading up to their child's birth. This includes eating well, getting enough exercise, and taking supplements during pregnancy. Many midwives actively encourage therapies such as acupuncture, homeopathy and massage for pregnant women.

Therapies in pregnancy

You may find that different therapies appeal to you at different stages of your pregnancy.

Aromatherapy

Aromatherapy uses scent to create a treatment that is therapeutic for both mind and body (it's a great addition to a massage as well).

Because aromatherapy oil is natural (the oils are extracted from flowers, leaves, seeds, herbs, bark and roots) there should be little-to-no side effects – but do choose your oil wisely as some are to be avoided during pregnancy and labour.

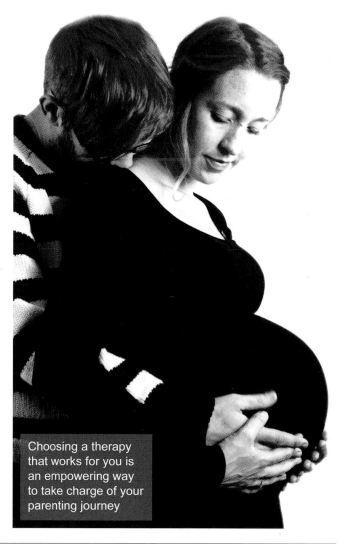

Choosing a therapy that works for you is an empowering way to take charge of your parenting journey

Sam: "During my third pregnancy, after a long day at work I would soak in a lavender-infused bath and lap up this amazing aroma. It helped my mind and body to feel more in balance. I still pop eight drops of lavender oil into my running bath now."

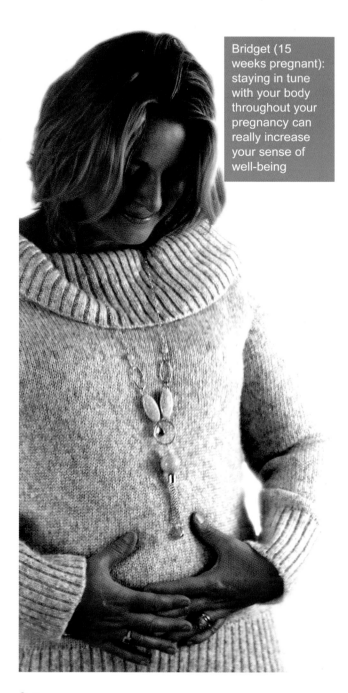

■ Essential oils

Essential oils are potent and highly concentrated, extracted from the very heart of the plant.

Organic is preferable; that way, you know that you are getting the best of the plant and no chemicals or pesticides will have weakened its healing properties.

■ The science behind aromatherapy

The term aromatherapy was coined by French chemist René-Maurice Gattefossé, who was interested in the aromatic qualities of essential oils. Having submerged his badly burnt arm in a vat of lavender oil, as there was no water to hand, he was astounded to discover that the burn healed far more quickly than expected, with no scarring. Gattefossé researched the qualities of essential oils and wrote a hugely popular book on the subject, *Gattefossé's Aromatherapy*, often called the first book on aromatherapy. (First published in 1937, it is now available in English.)

■ How does aromatherapy work?

The sense of smell is the only sense that connects directly to the emotional control centre of the brain, known as the limbic system.[8] Essential oils can be applied directly on the skin (usually diluted with a carrier oil), or inhaled using an oil burner or an electronic oil diffuser. You can also apply a few drops to your pillow or add some to a handkerchief to inhale. Essential oils should never be swallowed.

Many doulas and midwives promote the use of essential oils during childbirth, and many women have gone through labour with only aromatherapy as a means of pain relief. Doulas give support and advice to women through pregnancy, birth and the early days of parenthood. Filling a role that new mothers and families have always needed, they listen and do not judge. We highly recommend a doula if your support network is limited.

Our skin is the largest organ we have and is also permeable to a degree. When placed directly on the skin, the active natural chemicals of essential oils penetrate the skin through hair follicles and sweat glands. Artificial oils and lotions are made of larger molecules and simply sit on the skin's surface. Because essential oils are among the few types of matter that can be properly absorbed by the skin, they can work at a deep level.

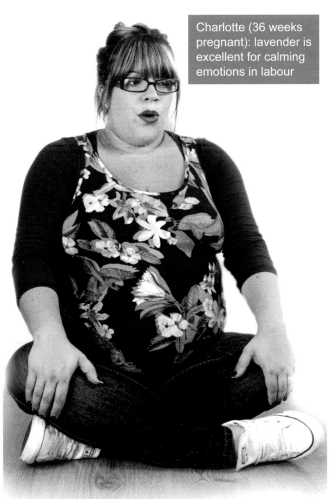

Charlotte (36 weeks pregnant): lavender is excellent for calming emotions in labour

■ The effects of essential oils

Each essential oil has its own set of properties that can help with a number of physiological and psychological conditions. The table below gives you an overview of some of the best oils for pregnancy and labour.

Please take care when using essential oils. Blending your own oils is a lovely hobby, but it is advisable not to dabble with unfamiliar oils during pregnancy. Follow our instructions for the safe use of aromatherapy.

Oil	Benefits
Bergamot	Antiseptic, antidepressant, refreshing, useful for battling cystitis
Cypress (to only be used after 20 weeks)	Antiseptic, diuretic, great for varicose veins, swollen ankles and haemorrhoids
Eucalyptus	Antiseptic, antibiotic, analgesic, antiviral, useful for clearing respiratory congestion
Frankincense	Antiseptic, sedative, astringent
Geranium (to only be used after 20 weeks)	Antiseptic, antidepressant, uplifting, good for muscle aches and poor circulation

Grapefruit	Antibiotic, antidepressant, analgesic, relaxing, eases fluid retention
Lavender	Antiseptic, antibiotic, antidepressant, eases fluid retention and soothes pregnancy aches
Lemon	Antiseptic, antifungal, stimulant, great for morning sickness and varicose veins
Mandarin	A relaxant, this oil is refreshing, and eases fluid retention in ankles and legs
Neroli	Antiseptic, antidepressant, antispasmodic, excellent at promoting skin cell regeneration
Patchouli	Antiseptic, antidepressant, nerve sedative, helps with indecision and confusion
Petitgrain	Antiseptic, antidepressant, refreshing, sedative, amazing for pre- or postpartum depression

Essential oils (when diluted in carrier oil) are a great extra to add to your hospital bag so that you can use them when you need them through labour. They can be a useful addition to a home birth. We'll talk more about this in our active birth chapter. The oils that have been found to make labour easiest are:

Oil	*Notes*
Geranium	In the third trimester this oil can be used to treat varicose veins and haemorrhoids. It can help keep you calm during labour, which is useful because anxiety can slow labour down. It is also good for exhaustion
Lavender	Lavender soothes uterine, back and leg pain, and headaches, and it can dull pain after labour. It is calming too, and when combined with coconut oil it can prevent stretchmark
Peppermint	If your baby is presenting in a posterior or breech

Holly: "It was only when I studied massage therapy and aromatherapy that I realized how much scientific grounding these disciplines have. Many people are under the misconception that because something is natural it is ineffective."

	position, try using peppermint oil. It can encourage the baby to move into a better position for birth
Rose	Rejuvenating for skin and tissue and excellent at softening ligaments, making birth that much easier
Ylang ylang	Lowers blood pressure and slows rapid breathing, making you feel calmer and more relaxed

Essential oils (when diluted in carrier oil) are a great addition to your hospital bag

Use 2 drops of essential oil for every teaspoon of carrier oil (or 10-12 drops per ounce of carrier oil).

Some oils should never be used in pregnancy as they have an emmenagogue action (meaning that they stimulate blood flow in the pelvic area and uterus, which can encourage dangerous menstrual bleeding). Here is a list of those that should be completely avoided during pregnancy:[9]

List of oils to be avoided during pregnancy

Angelica	Lovage
Aniseed	Marjoram (both Spanish and Sweet)
Basil	
Camphor	Myrrh
Cedarwood	Origanum
Cinnamon	Parsley
Clary sage	Peppermint
Clove	Rosemary
Fennel	Sage
Hyssop	Savory
Jasmine	Tarragon
Juniper	Thyme

(It is fine to eat moderate quantities of these herbs during your pregnancy as the potent properties will be greatly diluted.)

During pregnancy a woman's skin is more sensitive so it is worth being extra-vigilant when using citrus-based oils (such as bergamot, orange, lemon, grapefruit) as they can make your skin even more sensitive to UV light and may accelerate sunburn.

Massage therapy

Massage can be wonderfully effective at dealing with physical and emotional imbalances.

A relaxing massage can be particularly welcome in the later stages of pregnancy

A therapist trained in pregnancy massage will have more experience in positioning your body and ensuring that you are comfortable as well as safe.

Here are just some of the benefits of massage:[10]

- Tones muscles and increases flexibility
- Soothes sciatic pain
- Reduces swelling in the ankles (and hands and feet)
- Improves sleep patterns
- Eases muscle aches and cramps
- Increases blood flow, which means toxins are removed faster and nutrients are delivered to the baby more quickly
- Strengthens the immune system
- Helps to relieve anxiety
- Can work well during labour to reduce pain and stress.

Haseeb (3 months): massage benefits babies and children too; it releases oxytocin into the body, creating a feeling of well-being

Holly: "Pregnancy yoga increased my stamina so I was healthy and strong for the birth. The more in tune with your body you are, the more faith you will have in guiding your own labour. Pregnancy yoga classes can be an ideal way to meet like minded mums-to-be too."

Sam: "By the time I fell pregnant with my third child, I knew that consciously eating more nutritious food during pregnancy eases common ailments, improves your energy levels, and helps with your unborn baby's development."

Yoga

Many people have lost touch with their bodies. It is easy to forget that women are designed to give birth, and the changes that happen during pregnancy are all in preparation for the birth itself. Yoga is a great way to get back in touch with your natural instincts. Yoga creates a link between your body, mind and spirit, and facilitates real relaxation while getting you ready for labour. Prenatal yoga helps to tone and strengthen the pelvic floor and abdominal muscles.

You can safely practise yoga at home or attend a prenatal yoga class. It is advisable to tell your doctor or midwife if you are going to take yoga classes while pregnant.

Nutrition

What you eat and drink during pregnancy is important for your baby as well as yourself. Nutritional therapy is part science and part naturopathy (that is, a drug-free approach based on the theory that diseases can be successfully treated or prevented using methods such as diet, exercise and therapies). A nutritional therapist can give you advice that will help you with conception, pregnancy, birth and the early years of raising a child. A good diet can reduce stress and aid a good night's sleep, two vital factors for a new family.

Homeopathy

Homeopathy is the use of medicine from completely natural sources. Any plants and minerals used in homeopathic medicine are greatly diluted, making homeopathy safe for use in pregnancy [11] alongside conventional medicine. Here are some uses for pregnancy-related conditions:

Homeopathic medicine	Problem (s)
Arnica	Healing of bruises
Belladonna	Mastitis
Bellis perennis	Healing of internal bruises
Calendula	Healing of lacerations, grazes
Capsicum	Heartburn behind breastbone
Causticum	Heartburn with a craving for fizzy drinks and accompanied by vomiting

Hamamelis	Piles
Nux vomica	Morning sickness, flatulence, sensitive stomach
Phytolacca perennis	Cracked nipples
Sepia	Nausea caused by the sight or smell of food

Crab apple	Helps with accepting one's appearance
Impatiens	Reduces irritability due to inactivity
Mimulus	Helps to ease fears (useful at the end of pregnancy before labour starts)
Star of Bethlehem	Promotes a sense of calm after a difficult birth
Walnut	Helps one adjust to change

Heartburn is more common in pregnancy due to the rise in progesterone, which causes our muscles to relax, including those that form the oesophagus.

There is a fair amount of controversy surrounding homeopathy, but the one thing that people do agree on is that homeopathy is very gentle. The best way to decide if it is effective is to try it out, or ask friends about their experiences.

Flower essences

Flower essences come from distilled plants, and are a totally natural way to help balance your body, mind and spirit. They can be made into tinctures by adding a few drops to water and drunk. Here are some useful remedies for during and following pregnancy:

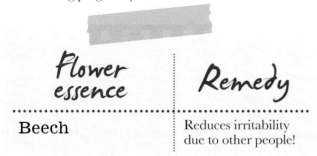

Flower essence	Remedy
Beech	Reduces irritability due to other people!

Reflexology

Reflexology has been used for many centuries. It works by stimulating reflex points on the hands and feet. Each reflex point corresponds to a major organ or part of the body. In a recent study, reflexology was shown to be highly effective as a form of pain relief.[12] Reflexology may improve your fertility pre-conception[13] and help to balance your mood before pregnancy. Reflexology has been known to regulate the menstrual cycle and improve healthy sperm production.

It can help keep hormones in check during pregnancy and ease fatigue, nausea, constipation, backaches and headaches.

It is not uncommon for women who go past their due date to turn to reflexology. Hospital inductions can result in a longer and more difficult labour; reflexology is a gentle way to encourage labour to start[14] and may even help reduce the length of your labour.[15]

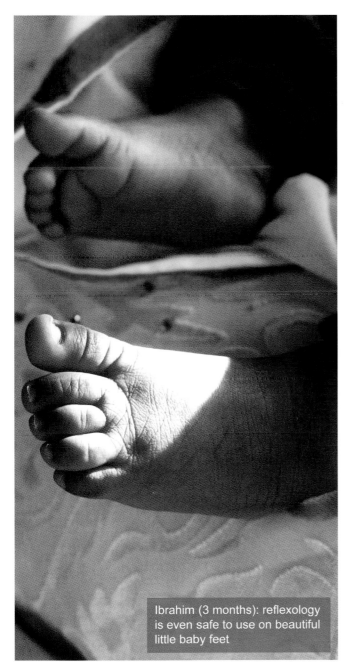

Ibrahim (3 months): reflexology is even safe to use on beautiful little baby feet

Acupuncture

Much like reflexology, acupuncture is an ancient practice that focuses on unblocking energy. Very fine needles are gently inserted along meridian lines by an experienced practitioner.

Acupuncture can offer pain relief, and has been used for centuries to treat some causes of infertility.[16] Many people also find it deeply relaxing and helpful in reducing stress.

Some are put off by idea of the needles used in acupuncture, but they are very fine and the application is superficial. You may like to try acupressure, which uses the same principle, but pressure is applied to the specific points instead (see the first trimester chapter).

Natural skincare

Pregnancy changes your skin, with hormones making it greasier or even drier than normal. You should try to avoid anything that contains parabens, sulphates or phthalates.

Sodium lauryl sulphate, which may be in your everyday bath wash, started life as an industrial garage-floor cleaner due to its efficiency at removing grease. Sodium lauryl sulphate, more commonly known as SLS, is an additive that allows your cleansing products to form bubbles. It's present in nearly all our shampoos, bubble baths and body washes. According to the Environmental Working Group's Cosmetics Database, SLS is a low to moderate hazard[17] that has been linked to cancer, neurotoxicity, organ toxicity, skin irritation and endocrine disruption.[18]

Parabens or benzoates are widely used in food and cosmetics to extend shelf life. However, questions have been asked regarding the safety of these preservatives. Women are starting to wonder if the rising increase of breast cancer is linked to paraben use. Parabens have been found in breast cancer tumours.[19] They have also been known to cause contact dermatitis when applied to damaged skin.[20]

Although pregnancy won't give you wrinkles, if your usual anti-ageing cream contains retinol then be aware that retinol may adversely affect your baby.[21] The risk of foetal malformation with oral retinoids is extremely high, even when used at a low dose or for a short time during pregnancy. All oral retinoids have an associated Pregnancy Prevention Programme (PPP), which is supported by educational material for prescribers, pharmacists and patients. Women of child-bearing potential should have pregnancy excluded before starting treatment.[22] Do some research to ensure that whatever it is you plan to use during pregnancy is safe.

Ingredients to avoid [23]

- Diazolidinyl urea (found in talc, soaps, shampoos, sunscreen and make-up)
- Imidazolidinyl urea (found in baby shampoos, bath products, fragrances, lotions and make-up)
- Diethanolamine or DEA (found in shampoos, cosmetics and pharmaceuticals)
- Triethanolamine or TEA (found in talc, lotions, shampoos and soaps)
- Parabens: butyl, ethyl, isobutyl, methyl and propyl (found in baby products, hair products, shampoos, deodorant, sunscreen, make-up and cleansers)
- Methylisothiazolinone (found in soaps, shampoos and bath products)
- Sodium lauryl sulphate (found in bubble baths, shampoos, soaps and toothpastes)
- Sodium laureth sulphate (found mostly in shampoos and baby shampoos)
- Synthetic colours (may be labelled as FD&C or D&C, followed by a colour and number, eg FD&C yellow 6, or numbered colours such as green 3, blue 1). Look for dyes derived from plants and herbs instead
- Synthetic fragrances (usually listed as fragrance or parfum). Opt for fragrance-free or unscented products, plant-based fragrances or anything certified organic.

There are some excellent natural organic skincare ranges available on the high street, like Mumma Loves Organics in the UK. We've included plenty of natural skincare recipes at the back of this book. Applying stretchmark lotion to your growing bump is also a wonderful way for you and your partner to bond with your little one before they are even born.

Holly: "I like to think that my emerging crow's feet are in part due to the power of giving birth and the delights and difficulties of being a parent. They are little indicators of our unique stories and I think we should wear them like warrior stripes. There is an honest beauty to a body that tells a story and has been on a journey."

David, father-to-be: "I was more than dubious when my partner suggested going to see a reflexologist to support her through the pregnancy and birth of our daughter. However, the reflexology was so effective; my wife seemed calmer and less anxious, plus her nausea cleared up practically overnight."

Natural Dad

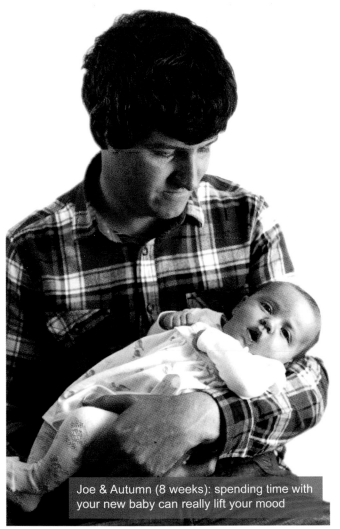

Joe & Autumn (8 weeks): spending time with your new baby can really lift your mood

One of you may favour complementary medicine more than the other. You may have your heart set on a natural parenting path, for example a home birth, while your partner feels a hospital birth would be safer.

Remember that complementary medicine complements conventional medicine, and is not intended to be a standalone practice.

Your partner will need to see a doctor, midwives, health visitors and perhaps even specialist consultants. She may choose to add a yoga teacher, homeopath, massage therapist, herbalist, nutritionist or aromatherapist to her list of experts to consult. If this is not financially viable, then there is plenty that you can do from home (including the remedies in this book).

With any aspect of parenting, the most important part is staying informed, listening, and then trusting your instinct. Collect as much information as you can and ask questions. Listen to the stories of friends and find out what worked for them and what didn't. Keep communication channels open between you and your partner.

Pregnancy takes a huge amount of trust for a father-to-be. Women are equipped with maternal instincts and hormones that will help them choose what to eat, when to rest, and what choices to make. Hormones are chemical messengers released from the endocrine glands that travel through the blood and have an effect on the nervous system. As a partner you can't control your partner's hormones, but you can be there to support and nurture her and your baby.

The father's hormones also play an important role in the parenting process. It has been shown that a live-in father's oxytocin levels rise towards the end of his mate's pregnancy, and when he spends significant amounts of time with his infant, oxytocin encourages him to become more involved.[24]

It is also important to address your own needs. Many men feel an overwhelming sense of responsibility and pressure to provide. Complementary therapies can treat all sorts of conditions including anxiety, insomnia and impotence and can help keep you strong and ready for the immense life changes that may be coming your way.

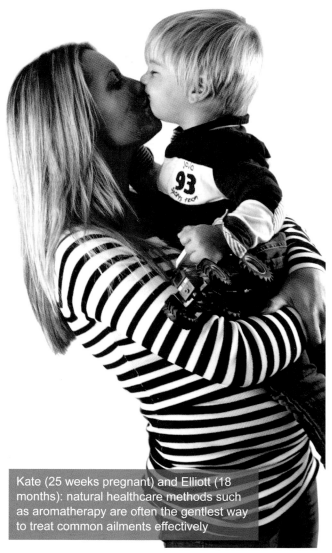

Kate (25 weeks pregnant) and Elliott (18 months): natural healthcare methods such as aromatherapy are often the gentlest way to treat common ailments effectively

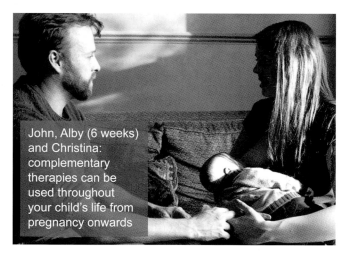

John, Alby (6 weeks) and Christina: complementary therapies can be used throughout your child's life from pregnancy onwards

Sam: "Pregnancy is the perfect time to get to know your body and your baby – and it's probably the only time you fall in love with somebody you haven't met yet."

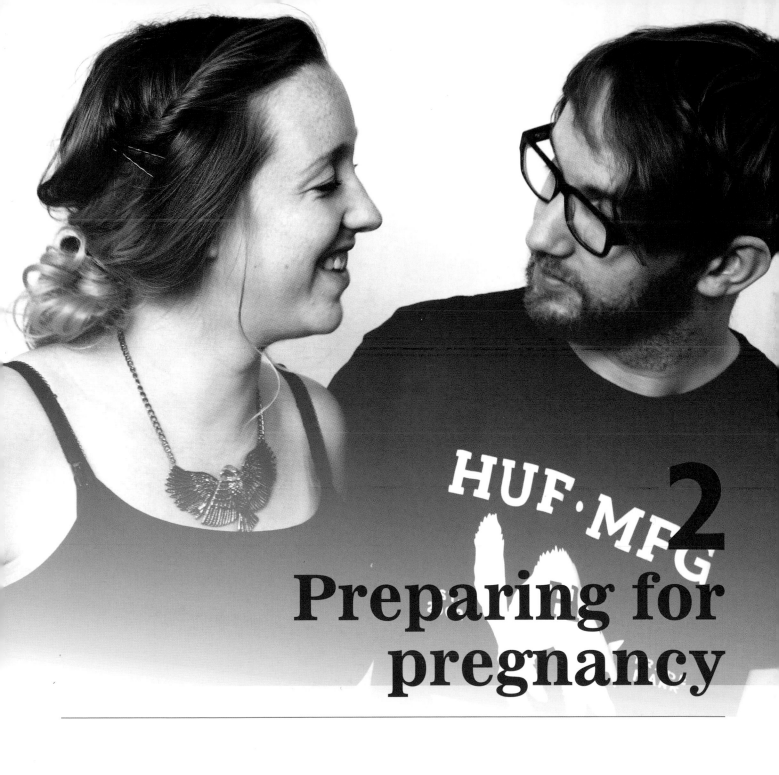

2

Preparing for pregnancy

2
Preparing for pregnancy

First, congratulations. If you are reading this chapter, you have probably decided that you want to have a child. The adventure that you are about to embark on can be utterly exhilarating and is, in our opinion, far more beautiful than any other.

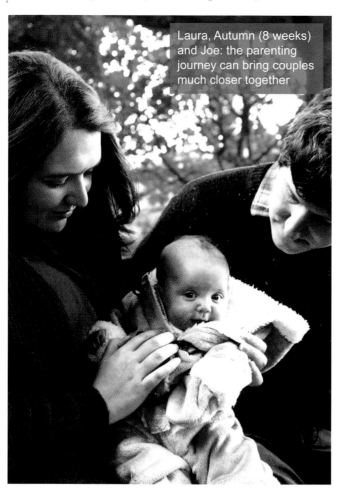

Laura, Autumn (8 weeks) and Joe: the parenting journey can bring couples much closer together

If you are already pregnant, feel free to skip this chapter and move on to the relevant trimester, where you'll find plenty of recipes, advice, tips, yoga stretches, and information that will help you and your baby to stay healthy throughout pregnancy, the birthing process, and beyond.

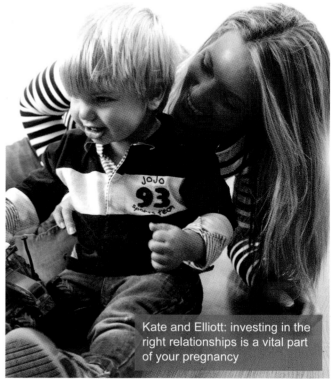

Kate and Elliott: investing in the right relationships is a vital part of your pregnancy

Talk it through

Deciding whether it is the right time to have a baby is a conversation that usually revolves around practical and financial issues. However, many couples neglect to consider if it is the right time emotionally.

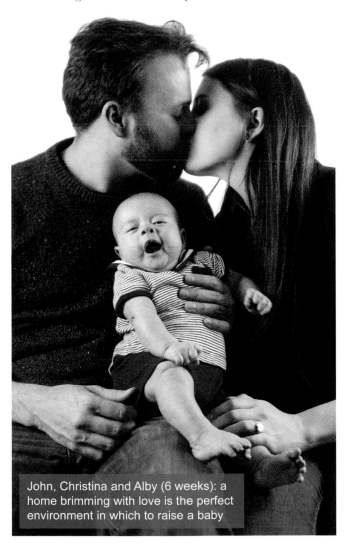

John, Christina and Alby (6 weeks): a home brimming with love is the perfect environment in which to raise a baby

Is your relationship as strong as it can be? The hormones produced during pregnancy can make even the most that are emotionally stable woman feel vulnerable and insecure. Many men feel obsolete once a baby is on the scene and most new parents struggle to find quality time together. You want to be able to use your individual qualities to complement the other's skills and to keep communication flowing. If there is anything that is playing on your mind, talk it through now. Parents who communicate well and listen compassionately to each other are more likely to give their children the balance that they will need to thrive.

If the conception was unexpected or if you conceived immediately with little time to prepare, then you can still use the duration of the pregnancy to connect and strengthen your bond with your partner.

Build stronger relationships

You might choose to use this time to reflect on all of the key relationships in your life. How will having a baby change your connection with each person? Are there any relationships that you would like to improve before your child is born?

The most important people to consider are any children you already have. Tell them how brilliant they will be as siblings, and share memories from your own childhood. There could be problems with friendships at school or self-confidence. It makes sense to reassure your existing children before another one comes on the scene. You could try introducing them to other babies or let them choose a special doll that they can care for. This can be a useful strategy later on while you are changing nappies and feeding the new baby.

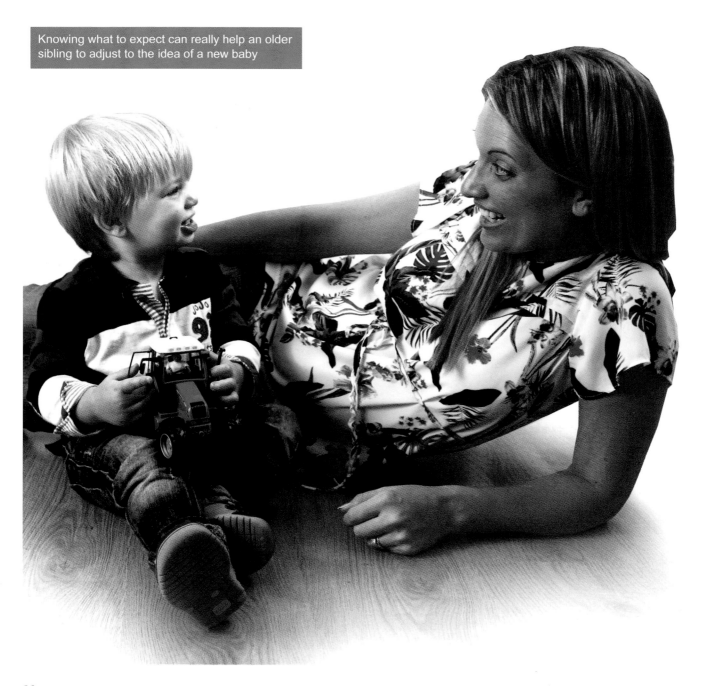

Knowing what to expect can really help an older sibling to adjust to the idea of a new baby

Consider other family members such as your parents. Is your relationship with them strong and open? Do you need to work through any difficulties? If there is a sibling with whom you have fallen out, this is the ideal time to take a fresh look at that relationship. Some stress in life is unavoidable, which is why it is so important to reduce the stressors that you can control. Pregnancy is the perfect opportunity to make a new start in many ways.

If you have any relationships that are draining your energy, this is the perfect time to create some distance. You won't have time for difficult people once the baby is born. Whether they are overly demanding, self-orientated, or make you feel bad about yourself, find a way to move away from them without confrontation. Block them on social media if necessary. Avoiding toxic people can ultimately feel very liberating and frees up more of your time to focus on the people with whom you have a healthy and, most importantly, a reciprocal relationship. Reciprocity is going to be even more important once your child is at school and you are developing a network of like-minded parents.

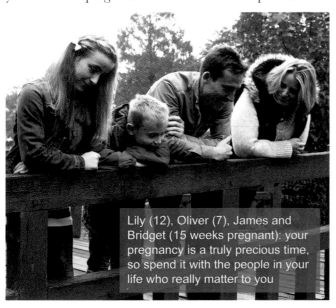

Lily (12), Oliver (7), James and Bridget (15 weeks pregnant): your pregnancy is a truly precious time, so spend it with the people in your life who really matter to you

Tackle your to-do list

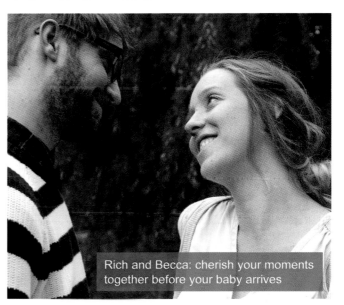

Rich and Becca: cherish your moments together before your baby arrives

Although this may seem the perfect time to tackle all the massive jobs that you keep putting off, you won't want to be doing anything too physical while you are pregnant (especially anything that involves paint fumes or heavy lifting) and you won't get time once you have a baby. Ideally, your home will be liveable for the next five years or so, without needing any major structural changes.

Do you want to pay off your credit card? Move house? Make the garden manageable? Go part-time? Research a more parent-friendly career? The maternity benefits of your current job may make it seem more appealing or you might start to consider a role with different hours or less physical demands. Make a list of all the things that you may struggle to do when you have a newborn, and schedule them in now. You can't predict how capable you'll be, so do as much as you can before you even conceive.

Plan some child-free adventures

No matter how many times they have heard about the demands of parenting, many new parents are shocked at just how all-consuming having a baby really is. The last thing we want to do is scare you off, but it really is worth relishing the calm before the baby storm.

If you are used to the freedom of going out for dinner, nipping to the gym before work, or even having a shower in peace, then do bear in mind that this is about to change. Once your little one is born it will be some time before you get a night out with your partner, an overnight stay, or a lazy Sunday morning together. Even popping to the shop for some milk can feel like a herculean mission with a newborn in tow. Things we take for granted like six hours of unbroken sleep, finishing a cup of tea and being able to wee without an audience become rare luxuries when you become a parent.

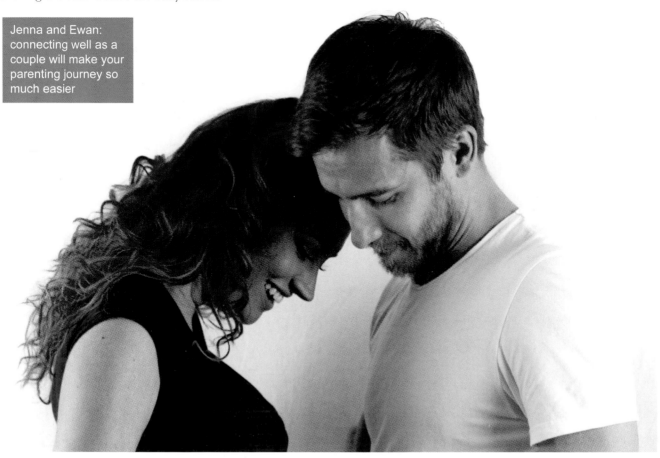

Jenna and Ewan: connecting well as a couple will make your parenting journey so much easier

Having a baby will take every last scrap of energy that you have, so make sure you get in plenty of couple time now. Book in lots of nights out and think about any burning ambitions that will be that much harder to achieve with a baby on the scene. So make a list of all the things that you want to do prior to conception and encourage your partner to do the same.

If you already have children, be sure to get some quality time in with them. Visit the places that won't be easy with a newborn, take them on a memorable holiday, or spend time doing what they enjoy most.

Get back into the swing of sex

So many long-term couples seem to have lost the knack of making love when they're trying to conceive. They are busy, they are tired, their libidos are waning. Suddenly having to have sex regularly because it is the right time can zap the romance and sensuality out of lovemaking. Re-igniting the passion that you had at the start of your relationship will help to ensure that making babies is a magical thing rather than a chore.

Oxytocin plays a crucial part in conception. This incredible hormone aids ejaculation as well as causing the tiny contractions that help the sperm to reach the egg. Oxytocin helps us to bond and to form deeper relationships, and can be increased by physical contact with people whom we care for deeply. This is why it is so important to focus on connecting and deepening your bond with each other (and not just during sex) during the conception process.

Oxytocin levels slowly rise through your pregnancy, peaking before labour and kick-starting your contractions.[1] Oxytocin causes your uterus to shrink after the birth and also promotes the let down reflex that enables the breasts to produce milk. This wonderful hormone that plays such an important part in helping you to bond with your newborn will also help you to bond with your baby's father.

Book in a weekend away (or a weekend at home without distractions), invest in some new underwear or dig out an outfit that makes you feel beautiful; share long candlelit dinners, romantic walks, and fantasies; bathe together, explore each other all over again. Let the sexual side of reproduction feel spontaneous and liberated. The more intimacy you share with your partner, the more in tune you will feel as parents.

If the physical intimacy has been waning for a while, break out the massage oil. Massage is a wonderful way of reconnecting without putting the focus on sex. It will also help to reduce stress, which is really important if you are hoping to conceive. In a recent study, a research team at Ohio State University in Columbus collected saliva samples from 373 women who were trying to conceive naturally.[2] The study identified levels of alpha-amylase (which indicates stress) in some of the couples. After a year of trying, 13 per cent of the women had been unable to conceive. Lynch discovered that the women with the highest alpha-amylase levels were twice as likely to be in the infertile group.

Sensual massage oil

5 tsp sweet almond oil (or grapeseed oil if either of you has a nut allergy)

3 drops of rose essential oil

2 drops of sandalwood essential oil

2 drops of ylang ylang essential oil

All three of these essential oils are known for their aphrodisiac properties. Rose also nurtures emotions, boosts confidence, and has an intoxicating femininity to it. Sandalwood is musky and deliciously sexy. Ylang ylang has a sweetness without being overbearing, and combines beautifully with the other scents.

The most important thing you can do is to look after each other. Value and respect your partner and take time out for yourself. The relationship that you have as a couple will influence how your children feel about relationships in general. (Even if you separate later, continuing to treat your ex-partner with courtesy and respect should substantially reduce the impact of your separation on your children.)

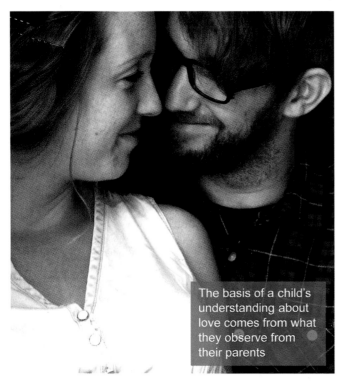

The basis of a child's understanding about love comes from what they observe from their parents

Health matters

Before you even consider conception it is worth ensuring that your body is in tip-top condition. The healthier you are before conception, the easier your pregnancy is likely to be.

Get into shape

The miracle of growing a whole new life in your body is a demanding one: your organs have to work harder (with much less space than usual), your stores of nutrients are being depleted and you are carrying more weight. In an ideal world, you'd be stronger and healthier than ever prior to conception. If you are overweight before pregnancy, then the extra baby weight won't only be tiring, but it can also make you more prone to high blood pressure and unstable blood sugar levels. Maternal obesity carries significant risks for the mother and unborn baby. Women of a BMI of 30 and over are more likely to suffer from gestational diabetes and to need an induction or emergency c-section,[3] and other problems can include pre-eclampsia, infection, and difficulties breastfeeding. It is not considered safe to diet during pregnancy, so try to lose excess weight before pregnancy if possible.[4]

If your BMI is less than 30, you may still want to shape up (visit the healthy weight calculator to check your BMI at www.nhs.uk/Tools/Pages/Healthyweightcalculator.aspx).

Sam: "When you're trying to conceive, there is no better time to shine the spotlight on your body and mind, and change what is currently not working for you with gentle exercise and an improved diet, while focusing on relationships and practical issues. But now is not the time to be embarking on a stressful new project."

Holly: "My husband and I practise yoga together each morning. It's a lovely bonding activity, strengthens my core and body, and keeps us relaxed and focused. Doing anything for your children (even those who don't exist yet!) is the best motivation to exercise of all."

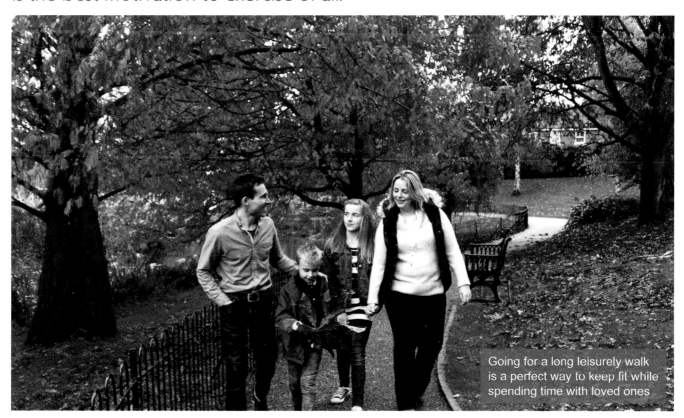

Going for a long leisurely walk is a perfect way to keep fit while spending time with loved ones

A BMI of 25 or above is considered overweight, so ideally you will have a BMI of 18.5-24.9 prior to conception. It is worth adopting a fitness routine at least three months prior to conceiving. Try to combine cardio, strength building and flexibility exercises. Ensure that you are consuming about 2,000 calories a day once you start trying for a baby. If your BMI is under 18.5, look at muscle-building exercises and ensure you are eating a balanced diet full of nutrients. Consider high-calorie nutritious foods such as peanut butter, which is high in good fats and protein. (Other great sources of protein are salmon, tuna and eggs.) Unsalted, raw nuts are perfect for adding healthy calories to your diet: try a handful of almonds, cashews, walnuts or Brazils for a high-energy nutritious snack.

Whatever your BMI, increase your intake to 2,200 calories during the final trimester. During the first trimester it is thought that your body relies on the stores that you had prior to pregnancy.[5] This is why it is so important to prepare for pregnancy and to eat a well-balanced diet before you conceive.

Revamp your diet

Many women find it much easier to eat a healthy, balanced diet when they are pregnant because they are focusing on their developing baby. Research shows that it takes three months for a new regime to become a habit, so start your super-healthy diet three months before you try to conceive.

Get into the habit of drinking about 2 litres (or 8 glasses) of water every day. This can seem daunting to start with, so it is worth reminding yourself that fruit teas count. There is also water in fresh fruit and vegetables. Although our bodies are brilliant at self-regulating, in pregnancy it is more important to ensure that you are getting enough water and you will know if you're not by the colour of your urine (pale is good; dark is a sign that you are not drinking enough). Water will help your organs to function properly, improve your skin, and flush out toxins. It can also help relieve morning sickness, enhance energy levels, and balance mood. Your developing baby will need water to grow, so start thinking now about how to get more water into your diet.

Try investing in a water filter and get into the habit of using it (and changing the cartridge regularly).

Eat plenty of vegetables and think about whether you can afford to go organic. Most supermarkets sell organic produce – some organic produce, like carrots, are surprisingly good value – and organic box schemes deliver straight to your door. You might even consider growing your own. Window boxes of salad greens and herbs work well for those without an outdoor space.

Iron is an important mineral for pregnant women, so leafy green vegetables are a must.

Iron deficiency is the most common nutrient deficiency in pregnancy. Iron helps shuttle oxygen to your cells, which explains why iron deficiency can cause fatigue, fuzzy thinking and lowered immunity.

Work out some tasty dinners that are easy to make yet brimming with nutrients for those days when you are too tired to cook. Fibre, calcium, protein, vitamins and minerals are all vital for your baby's development, so get into the habit of including them in your diet before you fall pregnant. This is a good time to limit the amount of fatty foods, processed foods and sugary snacks that you eat. A good rule of thumb is that if it doesn't nourish your body, you don't need it.

Consider supplements

Folic acid is heralded as the number one pregnancy vitamin because it plays such a vital part in the development of a healthy foetus. It can reduce the risks of neural tube defects (NTDs), so it really is essential. It is advised that women start taking it around 3 months before they start to conceive until the spine has formed (at 12 weeks). Folic acid is found in cereals, leafy green veg, brown bread and brown rice, but this can be hard to measure, so it's a good idea to take a daily folic acid supplement of 400 micrograms (μg or mcg).[6]

You may also want to take a multivitamin to support your healthy diet. There are a number of supplements on the market for women who are trying to conceive and during pregnancy.

Avoid chemicals

Some of the most common chemicals are found in alcohol, nicotine and drugs. Although alcohol leaves the body within a couple of days, getting into the habit of not drinking before you conceive is a good idea. Why not consider giving your body a break for a year? You might be surprised by how much better you sleep! With alcohol consumption being linked to changes in mood and behaviour, high blood pressure, stroke, hepatitis, cancer and weakened immunity [7] there are plenty of reasons for all of us to limit our alcohol consumption.

The Department of Health in the UK currently advises that women who are pregnant or planning to get pregnant should avoid alcohol altogether. Exposure to alcohol can cause an array of serious problems affecting a growing baby's spinal cord and brain. It can also lead to delays in developmental and cognitive skills once the baby is born. We support the Department of Health's advice that there is no 'safe' level of alcohol to drink when you are pregnant.[8]

Once alcohol is in your bloodstream it can reach your developing baby, so we would advise you to avoid alcohol completely during your pregnancy. Even one drink a day has been shown to have effects on the unborn baby.[9]

Alcohol is such a huge part of our social lives that many people really miss it when they are pregnant. We've concocted some tasty alternatives below.

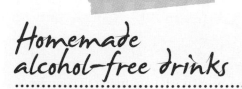

Homemade alcohol-free drinks

Ginger beer (also great for relieving morning sickness)

Grate a palm-sized piece of fresh root ginger into a saucepan.

Add the zest of 2 (thoroughly washed) unwaxed lemons.

Cut each lemon in half, and add the juice to the pan.

Add a cup of water.

Cover the pan and gently bring to the boil.

Leave the mixture to boil for 10 minutes before removing from the heat.

Stir in 2 tbsp of runny honey.

Add ½ tsp of cinnamon.

Mix together thoroughly and leave to cool.

Strain the mixture through a sieve and pour into a jug.

Top up with still or sparkling mineral water.

Add a handful of fresh mint leaves.

Serve over ice.

Safe rosé spritzer

Add a large handful each of blueberries, chopped strawberries and raspberries to a pan.

Add a cup of water.

Cover and boil for 10 minutes.

Remove from the heat and allow to cool.

Add to a blender with ice.

Blend until smooth.

Pour over a litre (35fl oz) of sparkling mineral water.

Watermelon ice

Cube a whole watermelon and blend it.

Add the juice of a fresh lime.

Add two handfuls of ice.

Add a large handful of roughly chopped mint leaves.

Include a handful of berries if you like – strawberries, raspberries, blueberries, currants and blackberries all work beautifully with the watermelon (if out of season, frozen berries are great too).

Research varies vastly regarding how long nicotine stays in the system. With this in mind, ideally you'll want to be smoke-free for a decent amount of time before trying for a baby. Stopping smoking is no easy task and it is important that you give yourself plenty of time to do it (see www.cancer.org/healthy/stayawayfromtobacco/guidetoquittingsmoking/guide-to-quitting-smoking-why-so-hard-to-quit).

Vapes and e-cigarettes are loaded with chemicals and should also be avoided. In one study, the flavouring chemical diacetyl was detected in the majority of e-cigarettes; this chemical has been linked to severe respiratory diseases.[10]

This is the ideal time for your partner to stop smoking too, not just for mutual support, but to limit the dangers of passive smoking, which can affect the child's birth weight, increase the risk of chest infections in the first five years,[11] and has been linked to Sudden Infant Death Syndrome (SIDS) or cot death.

One cigarette alone contains over 5,000 different chemicals.[12] These stay on clothes and soft furnishings, so even if your partner doesn't smoke around you, your baby may still be affected.[13]

Drugs (whether recreational or prescribed) can take up to a year to leave your system. It is worth talking to your doctor if you have any concerns about whether medication will still be in your system before trying to conceive. If you are on prescription medication, you will need to check whether you can take it throughout your pregnancy and if not, consider your other options.

It is worth noting that you can get pregnant very quickly after stopping any form of hormonal contraception.[14] Many women like to wait until they have had a period so that it is easier to determine a conception date, giving them a more accurate idea of the expected due date (EDD).

Some people believe that dyeing your hair during pregnancy can affect your unborn child and with a recent study stating that: "Alarming data points toward a link between hair-dye use in pregnancy and the development of several childhood malignancies in offspring"[15] it is certainly something to consider. The same study suggests that even those who dye their hair a month prior to conception can be affected.

Many hairdressers are wary of dyeing a pregnant client's hair as pregnancy hormones can cause dyes and colourants to act in an unpredictable manner. Your hair may react differently to colouring; changes in hormones can lead to changes in the absorbency of hair and even the hair quality so you may end up with patchy colour or a frizzy, unmanageable mane. If you choose to stop, you could use the period prior to conception to get your hair back to its natural colour or look for natural alternatives such as henna. There are plenty of chemical-free alternatives on the market if you want to keep the grey at bay. Look for products that don't contain p-phenylenediamine (PPD), ammonia, peroxide, parabens, resorcinol or propylene glycol. These products will be labelled as 100 per cent natural / chemical-free and a quick internet search will give you a variety of options.

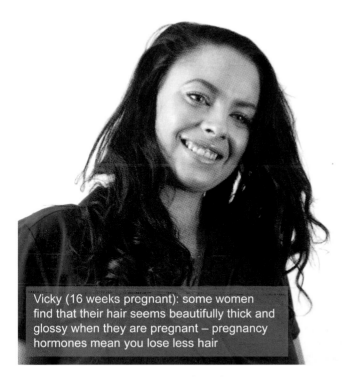

Vicky (16 weeks pregnant): some women find that their hair seems beautifully thick and glossy when they are pregnant – pregnancy hormones mean you lose less hair

a high-risk pregnancy. Even falling pregnant for the first time after the age of 35 can put you on the high-risk list, but as long as you are healthy to begin with there should be nothing to worry about. Women of all ages can have healthy babies. If you have other problems such as postural difficulties or backache, this may be worsened due to the immense pressure on your back during pregnancy. Think about strengthening your core with yoga or Pilates. These exercises can be done in a class or even via YouTube. If you have significant health problems, speak with your doctor and book a one-to-one with a trained fitness instructor.

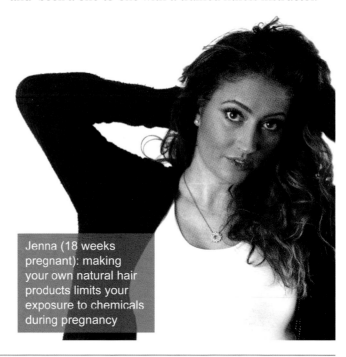

Jenna (18 weeks pregnant): making your own natural hair products limits your exposure to chemicals during pregnancy

Consider risks and health implications

If you have any health issues, factor these in before you get pregnant. Some pre-existing conditions such as high blood pressure, polycystic ovary syndrome, diabetes, kidney disease, autoimmune diseases, thyroid disorders, obesity, HIV and AIDS can put you in the category of

Holly: "When I had Jasmine I was a very healthy 19 year old. For future pregnancies I will be classed as high risk due to some surgery a few years ago. Being on the high-risk list means we get more medical support and we simply need to be a little more vigilant."

Mindfulness exercises

Mindfulness is the practice of being aware of this present moment. It takes you away from stresses of everyday life or needlessly reflecting on past difficulties and helps you to appreciate the present.

One-minute breathing exercise

- Find a space where you feel comfortable: lying down, upright on a chair, or standing. Set a timer for one minute
- Breathe slowly and deeply, filling your lungs and holding your breath for six seconds before slowly exhaling
- Keep this going in a rhythmic gentle manner. All you have to do is observe your breath as it flows through your body
- After a while you may find your mind wandering less
- Once you can manage a minute with ease then you could increase the time by thirty seconds or more.

Mindfulness walk

Mindfulness is all about awareness. Take a walk, making sure that it is a route you know well so you are not having to work out where to go next. Ideally, you don't want to go anywhere too busy. Walk slowly and steadily, breathe deeply as you go, and observe everything. Note how the breeze feels on your skin, the sunshine on your face; be aware of every sound, every smell, and every sight. Instead of filling your mind with your usual concerns, listen to the world around you.

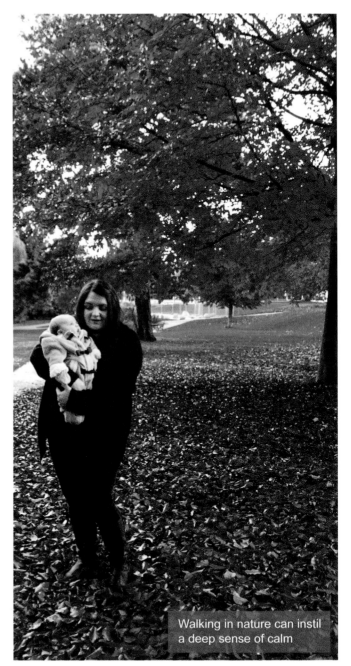

Walking in nature can instil a deep sense of calm

You can practise mindful walking throughout pregnancy, and can carry on after the birth with your baby in their buggy or sling. Walking is gentle and perfect for keeping you active.

Counting to ten

This is harder than you'd imagine. Settle yourself in a comfortable sitting or lying position, gently close your eyes and breathe deeply and slowly. Place your hands on top of each other in your lap, or on your thighs. If you are seated, be sure that your feet are in contact with the floor. Slowly count from one to ten, only focusing on the numbers. Once you reach ten, start back at one. If your mind starts to waver, return to one again.

This is a lovely way to find your inner sense of calm. It can be used during blood tests, internal examinations or in any potentially unsettling situation.

Breath is our life force and deep breathing is a wonderful way to get plenty of oxygen through to your little one during pregnancy.

If you can practise mindfulness, deep breathing and relaxation techniques, then by the time it comes to giving birth you will be very good at relaxing yourself deeply, using mindfulness to move away from physical discomfort. Breathing deeply will also give you energy during the labour, oxygenating your muscles to make them more powerful.

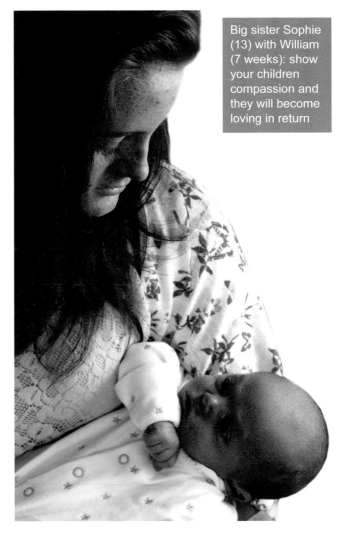

Big sister Sophie (13) with William (7 weeks): show your children compassion and they will become loving in return

Sam: "If you are stressed and anxious, your body will be working overtime in all the wrong ways. Lots of women find that once they regularly try to clear their minds, any fertility issues become a thing of the past. So if you are feeling stressed about conceiving, take steps to relax."

For the next three months prior to conception focus on

- Cutting out caffeine (or cutting back to the recommended guidelines)
- Limiting chemicals (and consider making your own skincare products)
- Drinking more water
- Reaching a healthy weight
- Building relationships
- Building your core (using yoga)
- Improving your diet and increasing your intake of nutrients
- Embarking on an exercise regime
- Preparing your home, your life and your body for pregnancy and beyond.

Parenting styles and advice may differ vastly, but the majority of parents want what is best for their children. Practising good self-care is vital to this, because if you aren't looking after yourself properly then you may struggle to provide consistently good care for your child.

By taking steps to look after yourself from the very beginning, you are ensuring that your child will have the best possible start in life.

Natural Dad

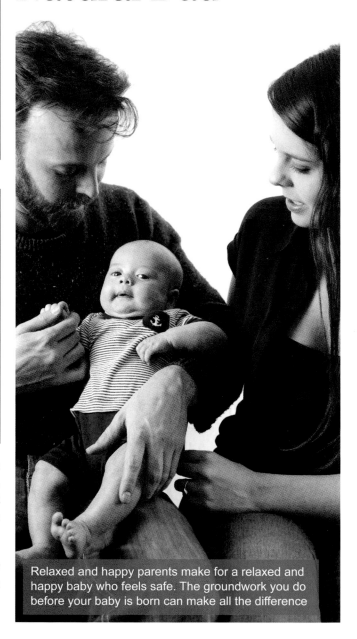

Relaxed and happy parents make for a relaxed and happy baby who feels safe. The groundwork you do before your baby is born can make all the difference

Many men feel the pressure to provide. When your partner is pregnant it is likely that you are going to become the sole breadwinner for a while, which can put a lot of pressure on you. Some men enjoy the challenge and it helps them to focus while their other half prepares their body for pregnancy. Other men worry that they are not up to scratch.

Sometimes men feel unable to discuss their worries because their partner is doing the lion's share by physically growing the child. This can be the start of a growing wedge between you. The demands of having a newborn, the steep learning curve of parenting, the sleepless nights, new financial pressures, and ongoing exhaustion can be a testing time for any couple and so it is vitally important that you are able to talk things through.

The best thing that you can give your child-to-be is your time (along with your love and kindness), so don't opt for a job that means you will rarely be at home. You are becoming your child's role model, which is more important than a hefty pay cheque. In the ideal world you would have a fulfilling career you are proud of, that allows plenty of time to be around for your children, and leaves you feeling energized at the end of the day. In reality, most of us make compromises once we become parents.

Consider the possibility of becoming a stay-at-home dad. Your partner may want to return to work once your child is born, and you may not even know what you want to do until after they arrive. The further you get along the parenting journey, the more you will realize the importance of dancing to your own drum beat.

It is easy to see pregnancy as a balm for a difficult relationship, but going through pregnancy and parenting together can put immense pressure on a couple. It can deepen the bond into something magical, but any areas of discontentment are likely to be magnified once there is a little life to take care of. Use this preparation time to share your fears as well as your hopes.

There is an outdated assumption that men love the pre-conception period because the focus is on having as much sex as possible. If you feel like your partner is too fixated on ovulation dates, try to guide her towards more spontaneous lovemaking. Just because you both want to conceive does not mean that you will always feel in the mood. Make love as much as possible without focusing on the calendar, as pressure can take the magic out of the act. If the process is making you stressed, then you may like to try some massage, meditation, a weekend away or a special night out together.

These months may also be the last period when it is just you and your partner, or the two of you and any older children. Take advantage of this special time together and weave some magical memories before the unpredictability of pregnancy.

Rory, dad to Ella, 3 and Jonah, 1: "If getting married was our public display of love, then choosing to create a life together felt like the most intimate way to show our devotion. It also got us both to really think about our health, and what we wanted to fundamentally change in our lives."

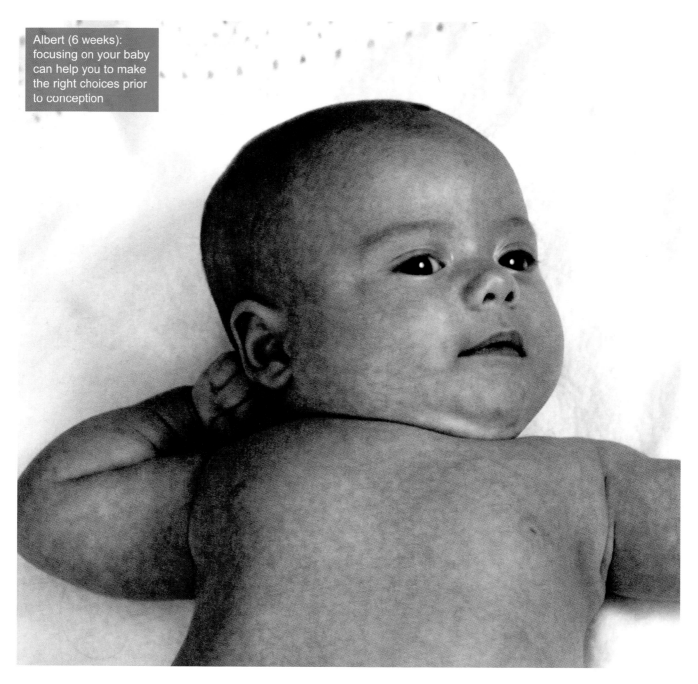

Albert (6 weeks):
focusing on your baby
can help you to make
the right choices prior
to conception

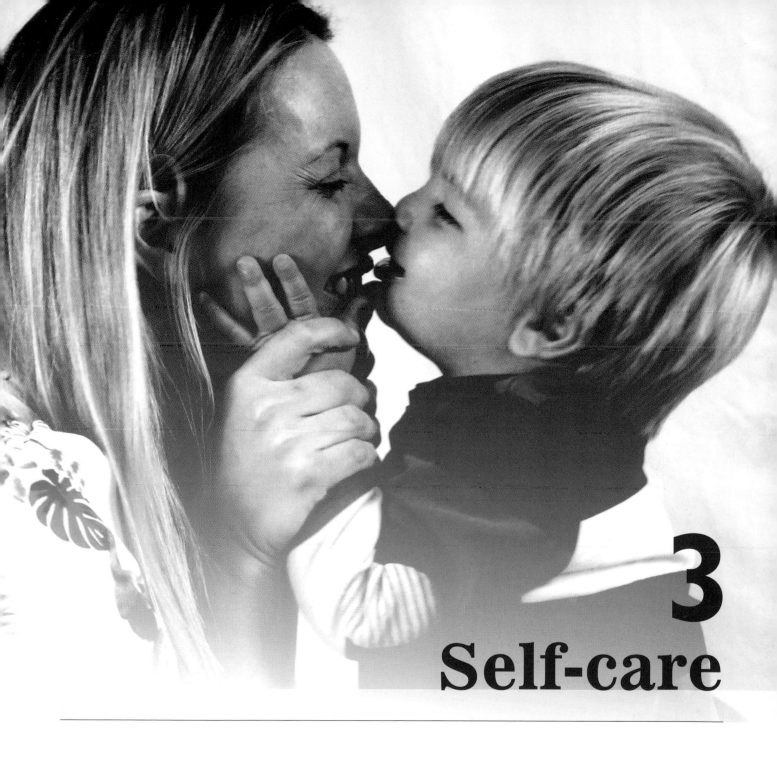

**3
Self-care**

3
Self-care

Academically you might understand the concept of sleepless nights, putting another tiny human first, and giving up your freedom, but in reality it can be quite a shock to the system! Pregnancy can be emotionally and physically exhausting. You may feel as if it depletes everything you have. You then have to cope with childbirth, an experience that can consume the same amount of energy as it takes to run a marathon (without the training).[1]

Without time to recover you are then handed a tiny being who will rely on you for everything. You will be more tired than you ever believed possible. You may also feel more jubilant than ever before. The love that you will feel for your baby is likely to feel like nothing you have ever experienced.

Self-care is something that we should all practise, not just through pregnancy and during the postnatal period. How can you give everything you need to the ones you love, if you are not looking after yourself? Getting to grips with the idea of self-care is so important in pregnancy, and we hope that you will continue to practise it throughout your life. In turn, we hope that your children will learn to practise it as they grow up.

Caring for someone else for the first time

If you haven't ever had to care for another person before, becoming a parent can feel quite overwhelming. Putting someone else's needs before your own, feeling that you are constantly on call, can be absolutely momentous. Spending time choosing an outfit from your wardrobe, blow-drying your hair or lounging in the bath can feel like an impossibility once there are children on the scene. Before you had a baby you'd be able to call in sick or cancel commitments. With a new baby, there are no sick days. There is no time or space for respite.

Sam: "I wasn't prepared for just how tired I felt after giving birth. After having my third child I didn't get out of my pyjamas for two weeks. Initially, I felt guilty but I soon realized this was just what we needed to do to bond and recover."

You might like to enjoy the last few months without a baby by focusing on your own needs, or you might consider that caring for others could be worthwhile preparation for when the baby arrives. As long as you stay away from places where you could contract illnesses or emotionally stressful situations (remember that your pregnancy hormones can make you feel extra-sensitive), helping out with an elderly neighbour or putting in a few hours at a local children's group could give you some valuable caring experience. Being around young babies might give you a better idea of what to expect when yours arrives.

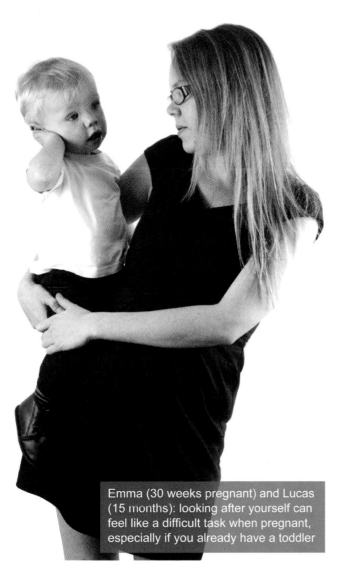

Emma (30 weeks pregnant) and Lucas (15 months): looking after yourself can feel like a difficult task when pregnant, especially if you already have a toddler

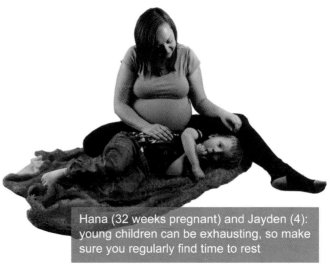

Hana (32 weeks pregnant) and Jayden (4): young children can be exhausting, so make sure you regularly find time to rest

Relying on others

Even the most fiercely independent people need to ask for help sometimes. If your partner is busy, then you might like to ask a friend or family member for help with key hospital appointments or anything involving heavy lifting. Finding reliable people who can support you in an emergency when your baby is tiny is vital. As your child grows up, it is important that they have adults whom they feel they can trust other than their parents.

So as your pregnancy develops, really relish those moments that you have to yourself. Each baby and child is different, so it is hard to predict how much pressure you will be under. Every time you sit down and enjoy a hot drink, or get time to be alone, remind yourself how grateful you are for this opportunity.

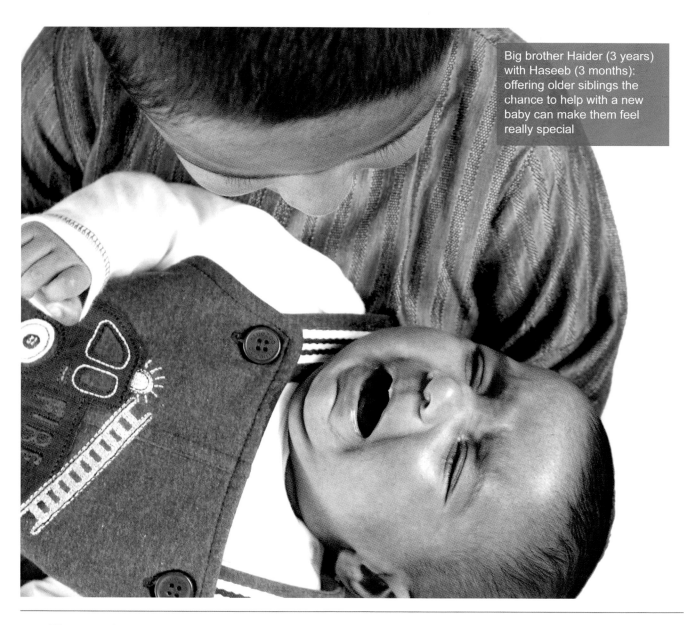

Big brother Haider (3 years) with Haseeb (3 months): offering older siblings the chance to help with a new baby can make them feel really special

Holly: "Independence is a wonderful thing but knowing when to seek support is crucial. When someone asks you to help them, it can be a real compliment."

Feeling alone

Not everyone has parents on whom they can rely. If your parents are no longer here, distant, or not well enough to help, then being a new parent can feel really difficult. Without available grandparents on tap it is imperative that you learn self-care and make it part of your daily routine.

For existing carers, the physical and emotional demands of pregnancy and parenting can be really taxing. If pregnancy leaves you zapped of energy, feeling sick, anaemic, or with problems such as pregnancy-related pelvic girdle pain (PPGP) or symphysis pubis dysfunction (SPD), then it is even more important that you ask for help. Your support network could include siblings, cousins or close friends.

The sandwich generation

More and more of us are part of the sandwich generation, responsible for caring for our own parents as well as our children. If possible, speak to your parents honestly about your concerns. No doubt they will be overjoyed at the prospect of grandchildren and won't wish to burden you, but if your parents have pressing care needs, you may find it difficult to distance yourself.

Other relatives may be able to assist you, or there may be local organizations that can help. Try to build a solid support network for your parents too from their friends, neighbours and extended family, and do involve local authorities, including your parents' doctor.

The medieval Levent proverb 'This too, shall pass' can be a useful reminder that life is fluid and always changing. Write it down and stick it somewhere crucial: next to where you answer the phone, above your desk, or next to the kettle. Talking to your partner about what you need is important too. Remind each other to practise good self-care.

Caring for the carer

You may already be caring for other family members or friends, neighbours, even your partner. This may make you feel as if you have drawn the short straw. Although your body knows how to grow your child, you will need to keep yourself hydrated and well fuelled with a balanced diet to reduce stress, and to rest whenever possible.

Stress triggers hormones such as adrenaline and cortisol, causing our heartbeat to increase and our blood pressure to rise, which will impact on our baby.[2]

Many of us have no choice but to experience stress in our lives, in which case we need to make time for mindfulness, gentle exercise and relaxation in order to combat the effects of stress.[3]

If caring is a part of your life that you cannot take a break from, then caring for yourself (and by proxy your unborn child) needs to be top of your list of priorities. Self-care has to happen on a daily basis. You need to rank your own needs as highly as the needs of those around you. A good introduction to this idea is to allow yourself five minutes every hour to do something relaxing or enjoyable; this could even be staring out of the window and losing yourself in your own thoughts.

Giving yourself permission

Many people struggle to practise self-care because it feels like an indulgence, lazy or selfish. They are so used to meeting the needs of others that they find it hard to value their own. Remember, to grow a healthy, happy baby you must nurture your own body and spirit. Your body needs far more than food and exercise to stay healthy and balanced. It needs rest and recovery time. It needs space.

The most important thing that you can do on your pregnancy journey is to give yourself permission. Go to the mirror, look yourself straight in the eye and tell yourself: 'I give myself the permission to look after my body and my mind, so that I can be the best person I can be for my baby. I give myself permission to ask for help when I need it. I give myself permission to take time out and to enjoy life.'

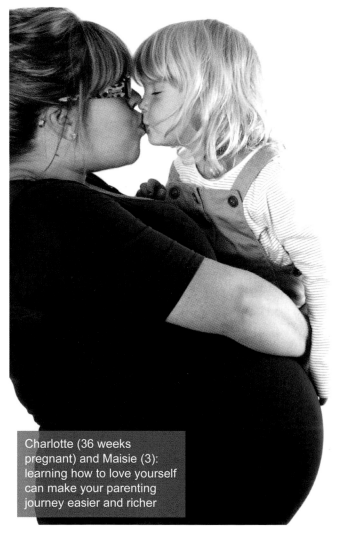

Charlotte (36 weeks pregnant) and Maisie (3): learning how to love yourself can make your parenting journey easier and richer

Making time

If you ask most people why they don't look after themselves, they will usually tell you that it is because they don't have the time. When you are a new parent, it can feel like you barely have two minutes to brush your teeth, let alone time to really connect with yourself.

In fact, you don't need a block of hours, or a whole evening, to do this. You simply need a few moments each day to devote to yourself. It may help to schedule it in. Really look at your daily commitments: is there anything non-essential that you can stop doing right now?

Pregnancy is the ideal time to cut back on anything that is not feeding your soul, or is not really important to you. Birth can be so much more than the birth of a child; it can be the birth of a whole new way of life for you and your family. Seize this opportunity with both hands. Trim away anything that feels superfluous and before anyone tries to fill in the spaces, think about what sort of self-care would work best for you. For example, listening to a relaxation tape, taking a long bath instead of a time-saving shower, or even allowing yourself to read a good book instead of cleaning the kitchen floor.

Daily self-care practices

Mindfulness

Mindfulness helps us to break the stress cycle and to connect with our hidden feelings and thoughts. Regular mindfulness can actually shrink the amygdala, the area of the brain that controls our fight or flight response.[4] This area is linked to stress, and if it shrinks the frontal cortex will grow. This is where decisions are made, and it is also responsible for concentration and awareness.[5]

As you read these words, push your feet into the ground, let each toe make contact with the floor and shift your weight around so that you are aware of the heaviness in your body. Just that simple act means that you are practising mindfulness. Building a better connection with your body is integral for preparing for childbirth. Believing in yourself and having confidence in your own power has helped so many women to give birth in a way that makes them feel in control.

Practising mindfulness in a chair

(This can be done at a desk, or in a sturdy dining-room chair.)

- You might like to set a reminder every hour, and just take a single minute to engage in some mindfulness

- Make sure your posture is relaxed yet alert, your shoulders relaxed, your feet firmly positioned on the floor. You could support your lower back with cushions, especially as the pregnancy develops

- Be aware of the weight of your feet and your back against the chair. Rest your hands in your lap

{cont}

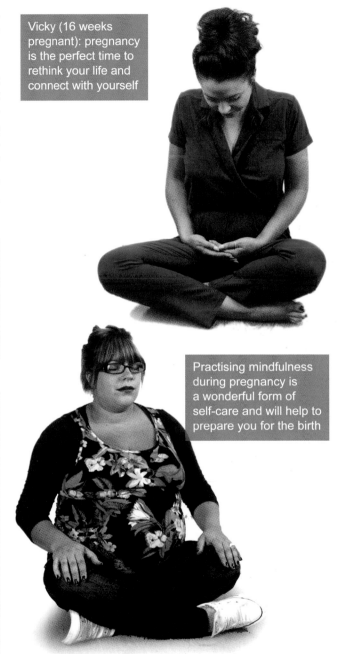

Vicky (16 weeks pregnant): pregnancy is the perfect time to rethink your life and connect with yourself

Practising mindfulness during pregnancy is a wonderful form of self-care and will help to prepare you for the birth

- Breathe deeply, inhaling through your nose and exhaling softly through your mouth

- Scan your body from your toes to your head, taking a few seconds to check in with each part of you – you may notice a feeling of discomfort or imbalance in certain areas. If so, just acknowledge the feeling and move on

- This practice will connect you with your body, help to release any tension that you are holding, and allow your mind a break from chattering thoughts.

It can also be helpful to engage in a full 10-minute mindfulness scan of your body each day. How does each part of you feel? This should be at a time that is free from distractions, or in bed as you prepare to sleep.

■ Mindful meals

Modern life is so starved of time for ourselves that even basic meal times often get rushed. Most of us have skipped meals, eaten at our desks, had dinner in front of the television, or snacked while we are on the move.

Preparing a home-cooked meal using mindfulness adds an element of ritual. Really focus on each ingredient, how it feels, how it smells, its colours. Enjoy the cool wash of water as you clean the vegetables, the pleasing bite of the knife as it cuts through each ingredient, the sounds and the aromas.

Lay the table with freshly cut flowers and beautiful linens, use crockery that delights the eye, play some music, add a special drink to complete the meal. When you sit down to eat, consciously engage with the food, savour each mouthful, taste the sunshine in the vegetables, and acknowledge the love in the preparation. Be aware that each mouthful is feeding you. Food that can be eaten with your hands allows you to connect with your meal in a different way.

Even if you practise the mindful meal just once a week, you are giving yourself permission to slow down.

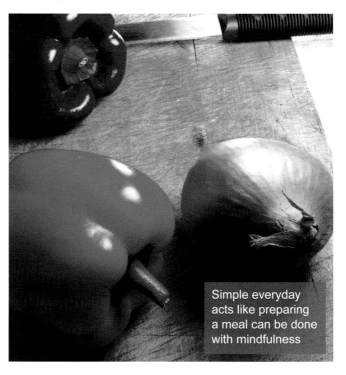

Simple everyday acts like preparing a meal can be done with mindfulness

Sam: "When I was pregnant with my third child I practised mindfulness while watching my older children play. Living in the present can create beautiful memories that last a lifetime."

Holly: "My workload revolves around different deadlines. I've learned that multi-tasking can stifle productivity, even though it makes you feel like you are getting more done at the time. Focusing on each task in turn will save you from burning out. Cultivating a calm mind will help you to function better at work, and make you feel more present as a parent."

Cut multi-tasking

Our meals are just one example of how we multi-task. We listen to audiobooks on car journeys, learn languages while we exercise, make phone calls on the way to work, and juggle emails and texts with our workload. When was the last time that you threw yourself into just one activity without trying to squeeze in other jobs along the way?

Constant multi-tasking can build more stress into your life. Can you practise yoga and just think about your breathing? Can you read your favourite poem or listen to a piece of music every day, and only focus on that? Can you stop juggling at work and tackle each task one at a time? Think of three things that you can do every day without distractions and commit to them. (It might help if you write these down.)

Journaling

Few of us make time for keeping a diary to note down our thoughts and feelings. Journaling not only allows you to explore your emotions, but also can help you to resolve any worries.

A pregnancy journal keeps track of each stage of your development, as well as your baby's. You might like to share this with your little one when they are older. (A pregnancy journal should be separate from your personal journal.)

A compliments journal can also be a very positive resource. You can either use a small notebook, or you could write each compliment you receive on a slip of paper and keep it in a jar or special box. This is a lovely way to focus on the blessings in your life.

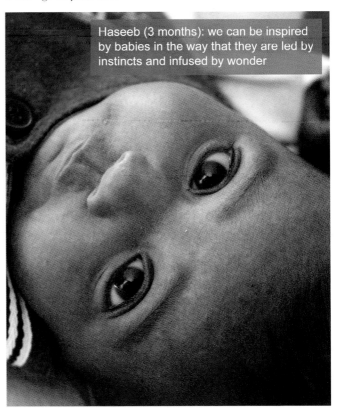
Haseeb (3 months): we can be inspired by babies in the way that they are led by instincts and infused by wonder

Wake up naturally

An important aspect of self-care is to get enough sleep. Listen to the signs that your body is giving you. If you feel like a nap, it probably means that your body needs extra rest to grow your baby. Allow yourself this time. Just 20 minutes may make you feel more rejuvenated.

Waking up naturally is not always an option when we have work commitments, other children, or a new baby to look after. However, waking up naturally is a good way to ensure that you are sleeping enough. Is there just one morning a week when you can sleep in? Maybe your partner could look after your children so that you can do this?

Ask yourself what you need each day

The most important part of self-care is giving yourself what you need. Do you need space for yourself? Do you need more sleep or a healthier diet? Do you need to see people who are inspiring? Do you need a break from stress? Do you need time to indulge in a creative activity? Do you need to laugh? Do you need a good weep? Do you need more exercise? Do you need more support from those around you? Do you need advice? Do you need to boost your self-esteem?

Every day when you wake up, really think about what you need right now. How will you achieve it? Do you need to ask for help?

Practising this element of self-care means that you need to look after yourself as you would care for a dear friend or relative. Sometimes it can help to imagine that you are your friend. If your friend was exhausted, would you offer to look after her children so she could nap? If so, ask someone you trust to take your children. If your friend needed to find a less stressful job, what would you do to help her? This is a great way to learn how to cherish yourself.

A huge part of self-care is knowing when to ask for help. Make a list of people whom you can rely on and give your permission to ask them when you really need support.

Unplug for an hour a day

The fast pace of modern life is exacerbated by the constant notifications, updates and demands that technology provides. We can be constantly on call. This can make us feel very under pressure so that we never fully have time to be in the present moment.

If possible, keep your phone on silent and check in at set times. Check your emails only twice or three times a day, perhaps after each meal.

Try unplugging your devices for an hour a day. You could even unplug your landline. Having one hour where no one can reach you could really help to relax you.

Take the time to go for a walk, have a relaxing bath, read a great book, listen to music, engage in some art, or focus

---

Sam: "Each of us receives messages from our body daily. It's important especially when you're pregnant to listen and to rest when you can. I wish I had listened to my body more in my first pregnancy."

on your yoga – without feeling guilty. Feeling rested is so important, especially when you are pregnant.

Deep breathing

We can practise deep breathing without breaking our routine or taking up precious time. Breathe in through your nose as fully as you can, hold the breath for three seconds and then exhale through your mouth. Doing this throughout the day can build up reserves of calm.

Self-date

If you could take yourself on a date, what would you do? Walk in your favourite wood? Read a book in a cosy café? Watch an old movie? Indulge in a home spa day? Write poetry, paint a picture, play an instrument? Create a scrapbook of photos? Bake something delicious, try a new recipe?

As your pregnancy progresses, find time every day to indulge in an activity that is purely for you. It could be for 20 minutes a day. Ideally, it will be an hour, but if you can only afford a few minutes try to schedule in a full session at the weekend. Write it in your diary, make sure it happens. Commit to it, as you would commit to a date with your partner or a close friend. If you find it hard to allow yourself this time, think of it as time with your unborn child.

After your baby is born, the idea of self-dates may feel impossible. This is where you need to go back to your list of people whom you can ask for help, even for just an hour or two a week. If your energy and resources are depleted, then you will have less to give to your baby.

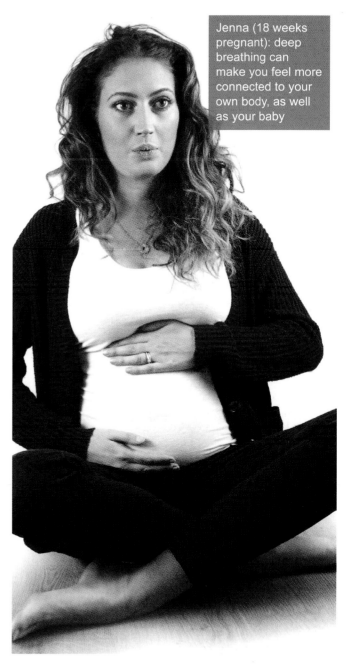

Jenna (18 weeks pregnant): deep breathing can make you feel more connected to your own body, as well as your baby

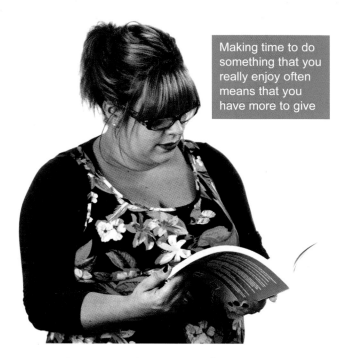

Making time to do something that you really enjoy often means that you have more to give

Looking after one another will deepen your relationship as a couple and your relationship with yourself. This will mean you have more to give your children, raising them in an environment where it is common practice to respect your own needs and the needs of the people around you.

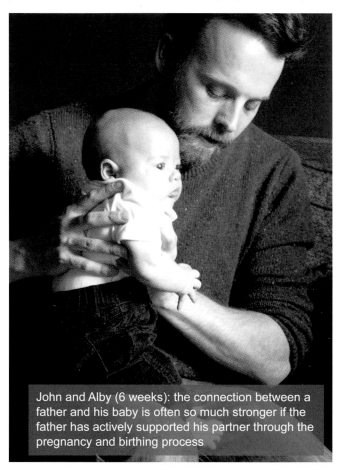

John and Alby (6 weeks): the connection between a father and his baby is often so much stronger if the father has actively supported his partner through the pregnancy and birthing process

Natural Dad

Give yourself the permission and the time to really embrace the concept of self-care, and try to practise mindfulness at work and at home.

Sometimes it can be difficult to ask for space, especially if your other half is feeling fragile. Perhaps you will each have your own space at home, somewhere where you go when you need to be alone. It could be the baby's room, a study, or you could decide that if one of you goes into a room and shuts the door then that is a sign they need some quiet time.

Nat, father to Wren and Lola: "I loved cooking for my partner when she was pregnant. I felt like I was nurturing her and our unborn child. Cooking also relaxed my mind after a hard day in the office."

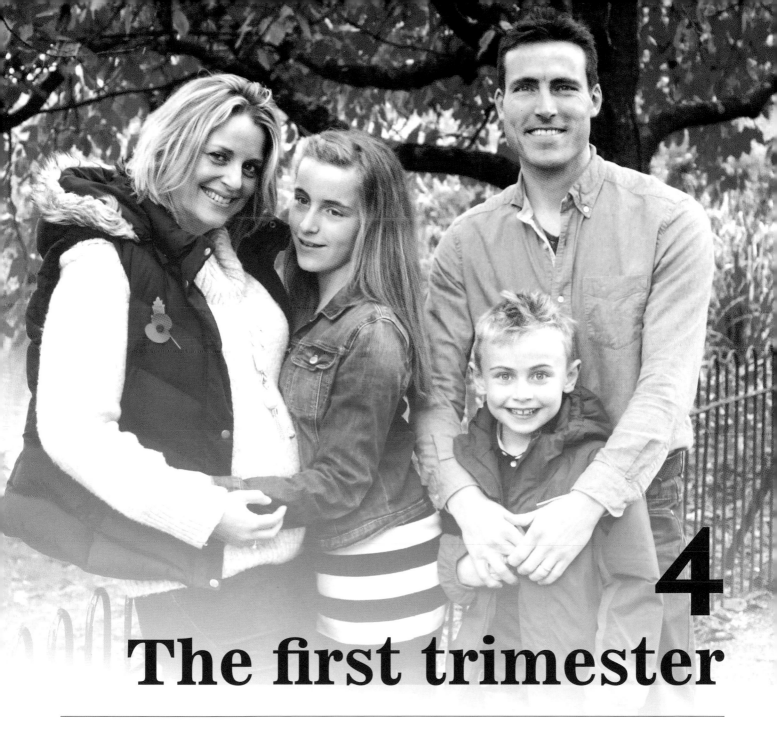

The first trimester

4

4
The first trimester

Finding out that you are pregnant can be the most amazing feeling in the world, but it can also feel a little overwhelming. Have faith in yourself, your body knows what it's doing; all you need to do is look after yourself (and by extension your baby) for the next nine months and the rest usually takes care of itself.

How your body changes

The first trimester is a time of significant changes in a woman's body. This starts with a dramatic rise in your levels of oestrogen and progesterone[1] which accounts for possible feelings of sickness in the early days.

A healthy, developing baby needs a healthy placenta in order to receive nutrients. This means that more blood is directed to the uterus. Maternal blood carries necessary nutrients to the unborn baby and removes waste products through pregnancy.[2] If you feel dizzy at any point, this is likely to do with your cardiovascular system.[3] Blood volume increases progressively during pregnancy, beginning in weeks six to eight. By the end of the third trimester, the amount of plasma in your body may have increased by an incredible 50 per cent.[4] Your doctor will check your blood pressure regularly, but you should tell them if you are feeling especially light-headed.

You will certainly notice an increasing need to wee. At the beginning this is down to hormones and the increase in blood volume (hormonal changes cause blood to flow more quickly through your kidneys, filling the bladder more often). Further on in the pregnancy the need to go is due to the fact that the uterus has grown, and is pressing on the bladder.[5] Despite the frequent urination, it is really important that you continue to drink plenty of fluids during your pregnancy. Not drinking enough could lead to infections, dehydration, and potential difficulties for both mother and unborn baby.

Another change in the first trimester is how you breathe. This is down to the extra progesterone produced during pregnancy, which affects the way oxygen is absorbed into your bloodstream. You're breathing at the same rate as you did before you conceived, but much more deeply each time, which may be why you feel breathless.[6]

You may notice the signs of pregnancy rhinitis too. High levels of the pregnancy hormones oestrogen and progesterone increase blood flow to all of your body's

Sam: "I often found myself on my feet at work when I was pregnant. I tried to avoid standing for long periods of time but if I had to stand, I kept my feet moving, which helped increase my circulation."

Sam: "When I was pregnant I found leaning forward while I went to the toilet was really beneficial. This helps to completely empty your bladder which means fewer trips to the toilet."

mucous membranes,[7] leading to a stuffy nose and flu-like symptoms. (There are a number of natural remedies later in this chapter.)

hyperemesis gravidarum, an acute pregnancy sickness that can require hospital treatment. If you're being sick most of the time and can't even keep water down, it's important to tell your midwife or doctor immediately.

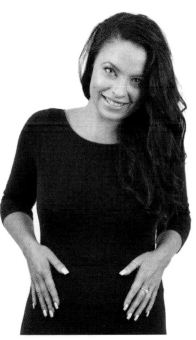

Vicky in the early stages of pregnancy: when few other people know about your pregnancy it can feel like a beautiful secret

Acupressure

You can try acupressure yourself to treat nausea.[8]

- From your inside left wrist, measure two thumb-widths towards your elbow with your index and middle finger. You should be able to feel two tendons. If not, wriggle your fingers around
- Press firmly on this spot, known as pericardium six: it's connected to the lining of the stomach and can help calm the mind.

Morning sickness

Morning sickness affects around half of pregnant women and usually lasts for the first trimester.

Morning sickness generally abates at round the 12-week mark, as the placenta has developed sufficiently to take over the work that the mother's body has been doing. If your sickness doesn't subside, you may have a case of

Natural ways to ease morning sickness

- **Vitamin B6**

The added hormones within the body during pregnancy combined with a lack of vitamin B6 are thought to cause nausea, so by topping up you can fight back.

Vitamin B6 is present in bananas, green beans, lentils, carrots, sweet potatoes, cauliflowers, nuts and fish.

▪ Nature's healers

Ginger and lemongrass tea

Ginger can be an effective remedy against nausea, and making your own natural ginger tea is really easy.

Add 4 cups of filtered water to a saucepan and bring to the boil.

Reduce the heat and add a large tsp of fresh grated root ginger and a stalk of lemongrass sliced lengthways.

Let the mixture simmer for 5 minutes before taking it off the heat.

Stir in the freshly squeezed juice of half a lemon.

Pour some into a mug and add honey to taste.

Cover the mixture and reheat it throughout the day for warm tea, or decant into a jar or bottle and place it in the fridge for a chilled alternative.

▪ Lemon

Lemons are so good at curtailing the symptoms of morning sickness that sometimes just the smell of them can stop nausea in its tracks. Squeeze a few drops into hot or cold water to sip (or pop in a slice).

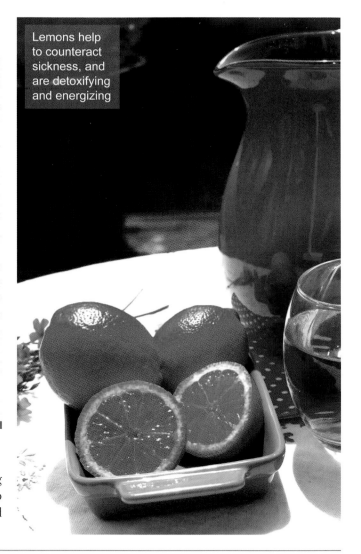

Lemons help to counteract sickness, and are detoxifying and energizing

Sam: "During my third pregnancy I suffered from hyperemesis gravidarum. I was signed off work eventually, but I still had two other children to look after. I used to make a batch of this tea and drink it chilled throughout the day. I sipped tea on the school run; it certainly helped settle my stomach."

Holly: "I inhaled ginger essential oil from tissues and sipped ginger beer, but the feeling of nausea was persistent. The sickness was worse in the morning, and aggravated by certain smells, tastes and motion. As soon as I hit 12 weeks, the nausea left. Keep reminding yourself that it won't last forever and try some home remedies to ease it."

Sickness soothers

Another portable way to ease morning sickness:

Heat a cup of honey (225ml / 8fl oz) to 150°C (300°F). This takes up to 10 minutes, and the best way to get it exactly right is to invest in a sugar thermometer. Keep stirring, and keep the heat on medium to low to prevent the honey from burning. If required, add a spoonful of butter.

Once you've reached the right temperature, leave to cool until it starts to thicken.

Add the following organic essential oils: 10 drops of peppermint, 7 drops of ginger, 3 drops of lemon, and mix together.

Place a sheet of baking paper on a baking tray and spoon the mixture on to it in lozenge-sized drops. You can use an ice-cube tray instead, but only fill a quarter of each mould or they may be too big to suck.

Allow to cool in the fridge.

Suck a soother when you feel nauseous. Wrap some individually in grease proof paper for when you are on the move.

▪ Rests

Sometimes going to bed and sleeping it off makes all the difference to morning sickness. Aim to rest whenever your body tells you it needs to.

If you find switching off difficult, try some meditation before you turn in, or gentle exercise. Just a light walk could be enough to help your body feel ready for sleep.

Dealing with exhaustion

You will get tired in pregnancy, and that's a fact. In the first 12 weeks or so, that tiredness may not feel like anything you've experienced before. Don't worry; during the second trimester your energy levels will most likely be up again, and you'll be feeling better in general.

As well as the flood of hormones and the energy it takes to grow a developing baby, often your sleep is disturbed because of a more frequent need to urinate, in addition to feelings of nausea, and this can all lead to exhaustion during the day.

Naps

It may seem like commonsense, but few pregnant women allow themselves time out for a little sleep in the day. If you can give yourself permission, you'll soon find that a quick nap is a great way to feel refreshed. Alternatively, get in the habit of going to bed an hour or two earlier than usual.

If sleep doesn't come easily, it might be time to try some essential oils such as a couple of drops of lavender on your pillow. Or research a better pillow! Some people swear by ethically sourced goosedown pillows.

Sam: "When you have other children it can be hard to rest especially if they're only toddlers themselves. I used to plan movie afternoons in the first trimester so I could take sneaky power naps."

Flower remedies

Olive is perfect for relieving feelings of exhaustion. Just place a few drops on your tongue throughout the day when you feel really worn out.

Activity

It may feel like the last thing you would want to do, and yet going for a walk or engaging in some gentle exercise (such as yoga) will give you more energy, and a surge in endorphins and dopamine, which should lift and stabilize your mood. Exercise will increase blood flow, helping your developing baby to get all the oxygen and nutrients that they need.

Just be careful of doing too much: take regular breaks and if you can feel your heart working too hard, or you become really short of breath, stop straight away.

Water

Being dehydrated can cause fatigue because your body goes into survival mode, and tries to conserve energy for an emergency. So ensuring that you get enough water during the day is essential. A good quantity to aim for is between six and eight glasses of water a day (more if you are exercising), but if this seems like a lot, bear in mind that you can also rehydrate your body by eating fruits (apples and oranges are especially high in water), vegetables, and even soup. Water can help with morning sickness too.

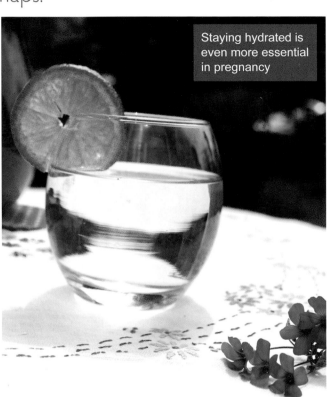

Staying hydrated is even more essential in pregnancy

Vegetables

Not only are vegetables a vital source of vitamins and minerals, but also they can help when it comes to easing pregnancy fatigue. Lack of iron can cause anaemia, which will make you feel exceptionally tired. Boost your iron levels by eating dark green veg. Not keen on your greens? Blackcurrants and apricots are also great sources of iron.

Natural ways to ease nasal stuffiness

Your body changes a lot during pregnancy so don't be surprised if you find your nose becoming blocked regularly. This is caused by the hormone progesterone, which can make the linings of your sinuses swell and become blocked.[9] Eventually, sinusitis can occur, meaning that you will start to get headaches and pains around the eyes and nose.

Keep your fluids up

Herbal teas and water break up congestion and help your throat to feel moist and comfortable.

Aromatherapy

Combine two drops of eucalyptus, lemon, lavender and tea-tree oils and add the mixture to a bowl of boiling water. Place the bowl on a flat surface and gently inhale the vapours. This will help keep your skin clear too, as many women find that pregnancy hormones alter the condition of their skin.

Vitamins

You can take vitamin tablets, but for a more natural alternative, good quantities of vitamin C are found in oranges, avocados, kiwis, dark green leafy veg, peppers and berries. Vitamin C is an important way to boost your immunity.

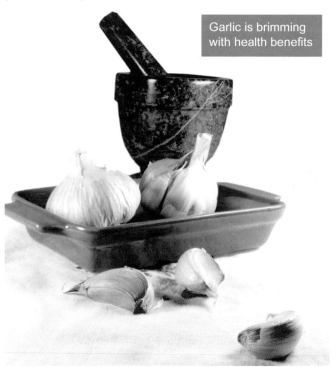

Garlic is brimming with health benefits

Holly: "I found that my body craved certain foods such as fresh mangoes and spinach. During the first trimester, I couldn't stomach cheese at all. Later on in the pregnancy my love of cheese returned. If you don't feel like eating certain foods, it is really important to look for the nutrients found in those particular foods elsewhere."

Garlic

Garlic also boosts the immune system, helps balance blood pressure and lowers cholesterol. Eating raw garlic may not appeal to everyone (although this is the best way to get the most benefits) so as an alternative you can mash the cloves and add them to an avocado, or make your own hummus. Olive oil, garlic and onion are a healthy flavoursome basis for any sauce.

Natural cold tonic

If the pregnancy rhinitis has been made worse by a cold, try this recipe to alleviate the symptoms. It includes cayenne pepper, which breaks up mucus; ginger, which boosts the immune system; honey, which is full of antibacterial properties; and apple cider vinegar, a natural antiseptic.

¼ tsp cayenne pepper

¼ tsp (ground) ginger

1 tbsp honey

1 tbsp apple cider vinegar

A dash of lemon (it helps soothe sore throats)

You can either drink this mixture neat, or place all the ingredients in a mug and top it up with boiling water to make a healthy cold-busting tea.

Taking it easy

Snuggling up on the sofa under a blanket allows your body to concentrate on resting, meaning that you should soon feel less congested.

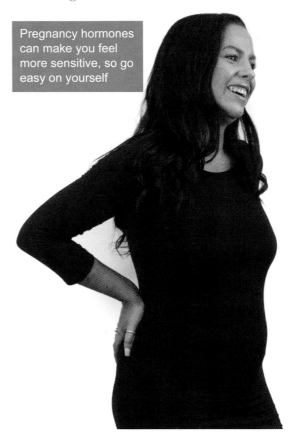

Pregnancy hormones can make you feel more sensitive, so go easy on yourself

Sam: "The first trimester can be a rollercoaster of hormones. I often found myself overly emotional and wasn't sure why. When this happened I would take time out to meditate, or if that wasn't possible, I would spend a minute or so in mindful contemplation. It really helped to calm my mind."

Holly: "If you are feeling particularly fragile, stay away from challenging people and situations. Nurture yourself, be open with your partner, and do what makes you feel good."

Changing moods

Moodswings and pregnancy are a very real combination and it is largely down to hormones. Sudden bursts of crying, anger, feeling sentimental, or being extremely sensitive are all par for the course. On a positive note, mothers-to-be become more empathetic with a heightened realization of the dangers associated with the day-to-day world, all of which will enable them to care for their child in the best way.

Emotional imbalances can make pregnancy difficult and becoming too caught up in a stressful situation can be unhealthy for mother and baby, causing heart and respiratory rates to rise. So take a look at these natural remedies to help keep your emotions in check.

Flower remedies

Problem	Remedy
Anger issues	Holly
Anxiety	Mimulus or red chestnut
Depression	Mustard
Moodswings	Scleranthus
Weepiness	Hornbeam

Mimulus is especially good when approaching labour as it deals with fears. If you are nervous of the pregnancy or the birth, mimulus will help you to feel more grounded.

Flower essence remedies can be bought from your local healthfood store and are available in many pharmacies. Add two drops from each of your chosen remedies to a 30ml (1fl oz) dropper bottle that contains mineral water, mix the contents and take four drops, four times a day. Otherwise, add two drops to a glass of water and sip at intervals throughout the day.

Yoga

Yoga boosts endorphin levels, reduces feelings of depression, keeps the body flexible and can increase maternal feelings through a release of bonding hormones. Yoga can actually make you happier. The 'love hormone' oxytocin helps you to relax and reduces blood pressure and cortisol levels.[10] Pregnancy yoga classes can be a great way to meet other mums. If money is tight, you can practise yoga at home.

Exercise in general stimulates endorphin production. When endorphin levels are high, we feel less pain and experience fewer negative moods.

Eating well

There are many foods that will boost your mood and help to balance hormone fluctuations. Dark chocolate can fight stress hormones such as cortisol, although try to restrict your intake to limit the sugar and fat content. Foods that are rich in serotonin include complex carbs and bananas. Omega-3s are linked to dopamine and serotonin production, giving us another reason to eat plenty of oily fish and nut oils.

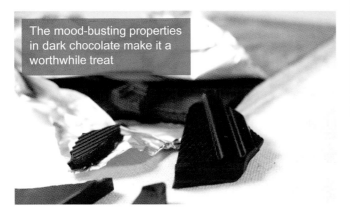

The mood-busting properties in dark chocolate make it a worthwhile treat

Meditation

Starting to meditate in the early stages of pregnancy will help your body and mind to adjust to all of the changes that are taking place. It can be invaluable once the baby is born too, keeping you centred during what can be an emotionally and physically draining time.

Visualization

Sit somewhere comfortable and close your eyes. Keep your spine tall, yet relaxed. Take deep, slow breaths and allow yourself to relax. It might help to rest a hand on your bump.

As you breathe, focus your thoughts on the baby inside you. Imagine what they are feeling, and how they are growing. How do they move? They must feel absolutely free within the warm amniotic fluid. What can they hear? Is it like the waves of the sea lapping on the shore?

Can they hear your heartbeat? It is possible to feel your baby's movements increase as you become more relaxed, almost as though they know that you want to connect with them.

You might like to try this visualization through each week of your pregnancy after reading about the developmental changes your baby is experiencing.

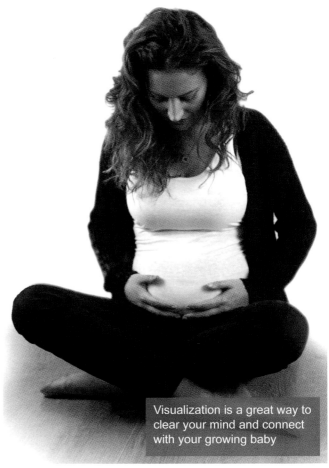

Visualization is a great way to clear your mind and connect with your growing baby

Nutrition in pregnancy

What you eat affects your baby, since food molecules pass from your bloodstream to theirs through the placenta.

You will need to avoid certain foods such as soft and blue-veined cheeses, pâté, undercooked meat and eggs, raw seafood, and liver. White tuna can be high in mercury, so it is best to limit the amount you eat each week to around 170g (6oz).[11]

Not sure of exactly what you need to see you through? Take a look at our handy checklist:

Protein

As a general rule, pregnant women will need about 80g (2¾oz) of protein each day. This reduces the risk of pre-eclampsia (and other complications), and it can lessen the symptoms of morning sickness. You can check the amount of protein in products on most food labels. When choosing your protein source, opt for leaner cuts of meat or low-fat cheeses to reduce the amount of saturated fat in your diet.

To increase your protein levels drink a glass of milk with breakfast and with snacks throughout the day. Try peanut butter on wholemeal toast for breakfast alongside a natural yoghurt, and some fresh fruit. Snack on nuts or cheese and biscuits. Eggs are a fantastic source of protein, as is fish and lean white meat. If you are vegetarian, then meat-substitutes like Quorn, which tend to be protein-rich products, can be a good option. Be sure to eat plenty of pulses (canned or dried), wholegrains (like brown rice) and legumes (like beans and alfalfa).

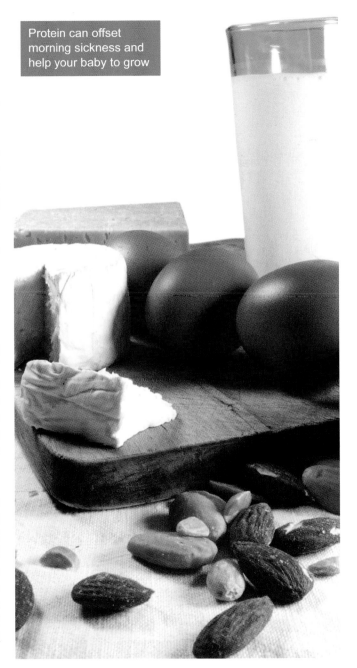

Protein can offset morning sickness and help your baby to grow

Fats

Healthy fats aid brain and organ development. Monounsaturated fats such as those found in avocados, olives, nuts and nut butters are really crucial, as are polyunsaturated fats such as those found in walnuts, flaxseed, oily fish, soya milk, tofu and seeds (especially sunflower, sesame and pumpkin seeds). Try to include at least one portion of each of these in your diet each day.

Fruit and veg

Fruit and veg should be a major part of every diet; they are packed with fibre, vitamins (kale, spinach and broccoli are all good sources of vitamin K, which helps blood clotting and builds strong bones) and minerals, and have a high water content. Aim to eat at least two servings of fruit or veg with each meal and snack on vegetable crudités or fruit portions through the day.

Water

Amniotic fluid depends on the fluids in our own body, giving us another reason to drink more water when pregnant.

Iron

Haemoglobin, the substance in your blood that carries oxygen around your body and ensures that your baby is getting enough oxygen, contains iron as one of its essential ingredients. Since you're sharing your iron levels (your baby could use up to one third of your iron during pregnancy) you need to make sure that your diet is rich in iron. Eating green, leafy vegetables like spinach and kale, munching on broccoli and seaweed, and enjoying seeds such as pumpkin seeds and black chia, will all increase your iron levels. Dried apricots, figs and prunes are a healthier option than refined sugar, when eaten in moderation.

Vitamin C

Vitamin C is a natural antibiotic so eating enough of it will help to prevent infection as well as boosting your immune system. It should be easy to get enough vitamin C – it's especially high in citrus fruits, blackcurrants, watermelon, strawberries, kiwis, raspberries, broccoli, potatoes and cabbage. Be sure to include plenty in your regular diet.

Folic acid

Folic acid (also known as vitamin B9) is very important for the development of a healthy foetus, as it can significantly reduce the risk of neural tube defects (NTDs) such as spina bifida.[12] Folic acid helps to ensure the iron is working in your body, builds red blood cells and enables the development of your baby's nervous system.[13] Root vegetables, dark leafy greens, mushrooms, salmon and orange juice are excellent ways to consume folic acid. As folic acid is so vital for your baby's development it is advisable to take a supplement. You will need to take 400 micrograms (μg or mcg) of folic acid during the first 12 weeks of pregnancy while your baby's spine is developing.

Vitamin D

Getting enough vitamin D is essential especially if you are pregnant throughout the long winter months of reduced daylight. To ensure that you are getting enough, take 10μg throughout your pregnancy. If you are breastfeeding, you will need to continue after the birth of your baby. Vitamin D is also found in oily fish such as salmon, trout and mackerel; mushrooms, egg yolks, and cheese.

Zinc

Zinc can help to prevent nausea, promotes growth, and quickens the healing process. You can find zinc in many foods including sunflower seeds, red meat and tomatoes.

Calcium

It is well known that calcium is perfect for growing strong bones and teeth. You may be surprised to know that it is also a natural tranquillizer, and therefore helps to keep you calm and ensures your nervous system functions as it should. Dairy products, sardines, sesame seeds (found in tahini), almonds and dark leafy greens are all rich sources of calcium.

B-complex vitamins

A general all-round useful vitamin. Getting the right amount of vitamin B will help your baby to develop (vitamin B is essential for development of the brain, heart and nervous system). Sources of this vitamin include wheatgerm, avocados, eggs and fish.

Omega-3s

Omega-3s ensure the brain (and the nervous system and retinas) develop properly. You can find omega-3s in hemp seeds, walnuts, oily fish such as mackerel and sardines, and rapeseed oil. This is a tasty substitute to olive oil and is readily available in supermarkets.

What to avoid

Caffeine

Similar advice is given by health authorities in the UK, USA, Canada, New Zealand and Australia regarding the safe level of caffeine in pregnancy as no more than 200mg a day. It is worth bearing in mind that high doses of caffeine intake during pregnancy increases the risk of miscarriage.[14]

How much caffeine?[15]

Espresso	47-75mg
Instant coffee	27-173mg
Latte or mocha	63-175mg
Tea	14-70mg
Green tea	24-45mg
Coca-Cola (can)	23-35mg
Diet Coke (can)	23-47mg

We would recommend trying to wean yourself off caffeine if you can as it's a stimulant with no nutritional value. Switching to herbal tea such as rose-hip or peppermint will increase your sense of well-being and promote good health (not to mention reducing tannin stains on your teeth!).

Processed foods

We all know that processed foods don't tend to have as much nutritional value as fresh foods. Take a look at the

Sam: "I used to be a coffee addict, but when I became pregnant even the smell of coffee made me feel sick. I was lucky I didn't want to drink it, as I'm not sure how my willpower would have coped with going cold turkey."

labels on some packaged processed foods and chances are that you won't recognize some of the ingredients. This is because some are actually not food. Processed foods may be more convenient, but the artificial chemicals used in some of them have carcinogenic properties. A University of Hawaii study of nearly 200,000 men and women found that those who consumed the most processed meats showed a 67 per cent increased risk of pancreatic cancer above those who consumed little processed meats. American Cancer Society researchers reported that a high consumption of processed meat over 10 years was associated with a 50 per cent increased risk in colon cancer.[16]

Our suggestion is to go organic when you can afford it and opt for home-cooked meals where possible: that way you will be able to enjoy fresh food throughout your pregnancy. Getting into the swing of creating healthy meals from scratch means you'll be a dab hand at cooking regularly for your children.

Bad fats

Above we extolled the virtues of getting the right amount of fat in your diet. As well as eating the right ones, it is also essential that you look out for the 'bad' ones. Saturated fats, found in butter and lard, pies, cakes and biscuits, fatty cuts of meat, sausages and bacon, cheese and cream,[17] can build up cholesterol levels over time, and have no nutritional value. Keeping your intake of saturated fats low will help prevent excess weight gain in pregnancy and reduce your risk of heart disease.

Sugar

Refined sugar provides us with empty calories and can make energy levels peak too quickly. We are better off with slow-burning energy sources that will keep us feeling alert for longer. Fructose is a natural sugar found in fruit and honey and is believed to be healthier than refined sugars. Swapping your honey to manuka honey could also enhance your health. Manuka honey is produced in New Zealand by bees that pollinate the native manuka bush and has powerful healing properties. Advocates say it treats many common ailments from soothing stomach upsets to healing eczema, as well as increasing immunity.[18]

Things to start doing in the first trimester
Pelvic-floor exercises

A strong pelvic floor isn't just about giving birth; it will also stop you leaking urine as the baby develops and pushes down on your bladder. A strong pelvic floor can increase

Holly: "Most people prefer not to announce their pregnancy until they are safely over the 12-week mark, but when I found out I was pregnant I wanted to tell the world. Is this an announcement you will want to share over social media? This will be the first of many choices you will make as you progress through your pregnancy."

sensitivity during sex and give you stronger orgasms. Keeping your pelvic-floor muscles toned throughout pregnancy and in the postnatal period can help with decreased vaginal sensitivity after the birth, and give you more control over your bladder. Get into the habit of practising your pelvic-floor exercises (or Kegels) regularly.

Kegels

- To locate your pelvic-floor muscles, imagine you are trying to stop weeing midstream
- Squeeze in sets of 10 throughout the day. You could do them as you watch TV, while you are sitting on the bus, when you queue in a shop, or even at your desk
- Every week, try to increase the length and number of the repetitions
- Keep these exercises going right through pregnancy and the postnatal period.

Reduce chemicals around the home

Get into the habit of wearing gloves during household chores and avoid chemicals where possible. If chemicals have been used, keep the area well ventilated.

- Try cleaning windows and glass with vinegar and newspaper for shiny, smear-free glass
- For a safe bathroom cleaner, combine ½ cup of white vinegar with ¼ cup of baking soda. For extra antibacterial properties and a pleasant scent, add 2 drops of tea-tree oil, 2 drops of lavender oil and 3 drops of tangerine essential oil

- Equal parts of lemon juice and olive oil can bring out the shine in unpolished wood. Apply with a soft cloth.

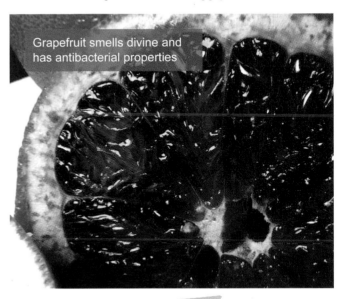
Grapefruit smells divine and has antibacterial properties

Homemade natural antibacterial home cleanser recipe

Peel a large grapefruit and place the peel in a glass jar with 2 cups of white vinegar. Seal the jar and leave in a dark place for a week. (Don't let any of the grapefruit flesh into the jar as it will spoil the vinegar. Instead eat it for an immunity-boosting treat!)

After a week the vinegar should have changed to a pleasing yellow shade and smell delicately citrusy. Sieve the liquid to remove the peel, and transfer it to a spray bottle.

Add 6 drops of tea-tree oil and shake gently.

Use around the house to keep surfaces clean and fight bacteria.

Learn to spot danger signs

Seek medical attention at the first signs of cramping and bleeding. Mild cramps can be your muscles stretching, but when they are accompanied by bleeding you need to take it seriously.

Nausea is common during pregnancy, but if you are struggling to eat or to keep down fluids then see your doctor. Dehydration in pregnancy can be very dangerous for mother and unborn baby.

Invest in a maternity bra

A properly fitted maternity bra will support your breasts and help to avoid backache as your bump grows. You will need to have regular fittings to ensure that your bra is suitable. Women grow at different rates during pregnancy, so there is no hard and fast rule as to how often you need to be fitted. Just be aware of your body and get fitted when you need to. At 36-38 weeks you'll want to invest in a nursing bra if you've decided to breastfeed, ready for your baby's arrival.

The developing baby – the first 12 weeks[19]

Week 1
The sperm and egg join together to form a zygote, which then makes its way to the uterus.

Week 2
The zygote is now called a blastocyst, and develops a hollow cavity in the centre. After approximately 72 hours in the uterus, the blastocyst 'implants' into the uterus wall.

Week 3
The blastocyst is around the size of a pinhead, but it is now growing at an incredible rate. The cells within the cavity are changing and becoming the embryo.

Week 4
The embryo has grown massively (although it is just 2mm/$\frac{1}{16}$" long, and weighing less than 1g/$\frac{1}{30}$oz). Hair, nails, teeth enamel, eye lenses, mammary glands, the inner ear, the nervous system, retina, muscles, blood, bone, cartilage, pituitary gland, lungs, trachea, lymph cells, pancreas, bladder and liver are all forming now. The coming 5 weeks are crucial to the baby's development. The gestational sac should now be visible on a transvaginal ultrasound.

Week 5
At just over a month, the heart begins to develop. Organs are developing fast, while the neural tube between the brain and spinal cord begins to fuse.

Week 6
Your baby is now the size of your fingertip, and their heart is racing along at around 180 beats per minute (twice the speed of yours). More human features are beginning to be recognizable; including eyelids, ears, and hands and feet.

Week 7
Your baby's arms and legs are developing and the nervous system is coming along nicely. Ultrasounds should be able to identify heart motion.

Week 8

Now you are carrying a foetus rather than an embryo, and that foetus is about 2.5cm (1") long. The umbilical cord is properly formed now. At this stage the baby will be able to open and close their mouth. The genitals also become male or female, although you cannot yet tell the baby's sex.

Week 9

Your baby is now around 4cm (1⅝") long. Their brain is already four times larger than it was at week 5 and the digestive system is almost fully formed.

Week 10

This is the point when your baby starts to looks like a baby! The amniotic sac is completely formed, and movements are more precise thanks to a mature nervous system. Eyelids will soon fuse over the eyes, closing them for the next 15 weeks.

Week 11

The liver and kidneys are now functioning, and your baby's head is growing larger in order to keep the brain safe. The baby will be around 5cm (2") now.

Week 12

Amazingly, although they are just 6cm (2½") long, your baby is fully formed.

Natural Dad

The first 12 weeks are full of emotions, joy, excitement and amazement but they can also feel a little daunting. It may take time to get your head around the idea that your partner is growing a whole other life inside her, a life that shares your DNA. Thinking that your partner has another heart beating inside her is a mindblowing concept. You might simply feel overwhelmed with the wonder of it all.

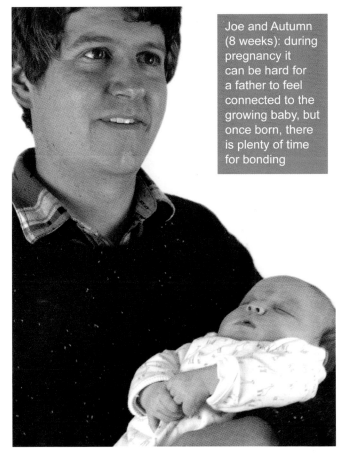

Joe and Autumn (8 weeks): during pregnancy it can be hard for a father to feel connected to the growing baby, but once born, there is plenty of time for bonding

Few people may know about the pregnancy; perhaps just you both and your partner's doctor. You may feel like your whole world is changing, and yet life outside your window continues as usual.

Your partner won't be showing just yet and so no one at her workplace will be treating her any differently, which might be quite challenging if she is suffering from exhaustion. You might find yourself doing more of the cooking, if certain smells are making her nauseous, or having to explore strange new recipes to suit your partner's changing palate and cravings.

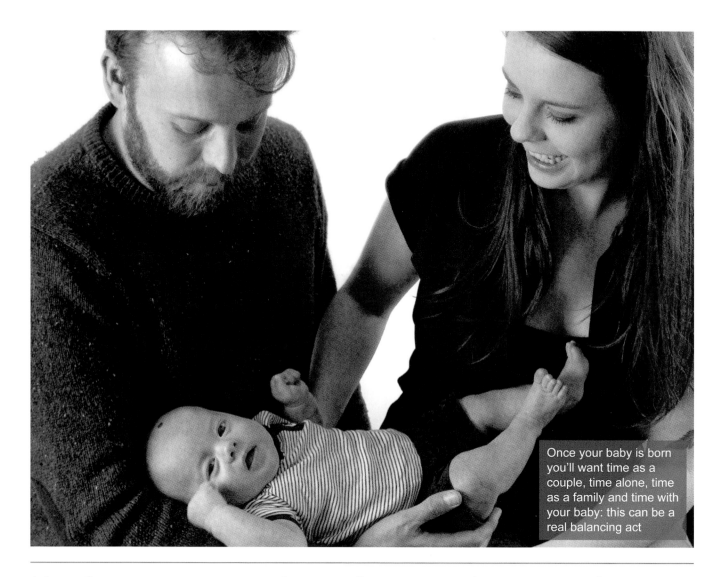

Once your baby is born you'll want time as a couple, time alone, time as a family and time with your baby: this can be a real balancing act

Manolo, partner to Lucie (24 weeks pregnant): "I was over the moon when I found out we were pregnant. We decided not to tell anyone, not even our parents, until after the first scan. Having our little secret brought us closer at what was a stressful time."

You may find yourself caring for your partner more than usual, especially if she is experiencing morning sickness, and you may be taking on more of a role with childcare, so it is even more vital that you look after yourself too. If you already have children, this is an important time to talk to them about what is happening with your partner. Showing your little ones how to care for your partner will encourage them to develop empathy, and help them to bond with the baby before it is even born. You may decide to let your toddler help make lunch, or make Mummy and baby a special card.

seed, at 5 weeks the size of a peppercorn, at 6 weeks the size of a kernel of sweetcorn, at 7 weeks the size of a pea, at 8 weeks a bean, at 9 weeks a cherry, at 10 weeks a prune, at 11 weeks a Brussels sprout, at 12 weeks a passion fruit. (This will introduce your children to new fruits too!)

Ways for little ones to feel included

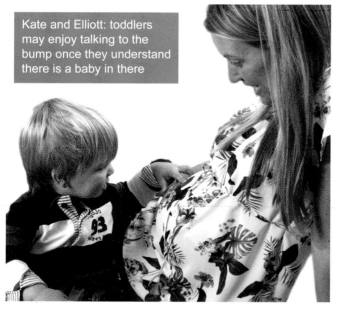

Kate and Elliott: toddlers may enjoy talking to the bump once they understand there is a baby in there

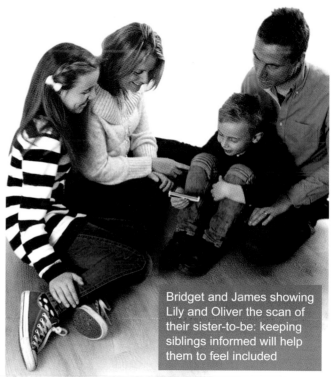

Bridget and James showing Lily and Oliver the scan of their sister-to-be: keeping siblings informed will help them to feel included

- Show siblings pictures of how a baby develops, week by week. Explain what is happening to the baby, which of its organs have developed, and how big it is. For example, at 4 weeks the baby will be the size of a poppy

- Get your little one to think about how the baby will look, and encourage them to draw pictures. How will your partner look next month? Can they paint a picture of the baby?

- Ask them to talk to the bump and tell their sibling-to-be about the world. Let them gently rub oil into the bump, using something high in linoleic acid that is suitable for delicate skin, like grapeseed oil. (Avoid nut oils in case of potential allergy.)

- Children can also give their mum a hand massage. Rather than giving specific instructions, let your child explore and see what feels nice

- As the bump progresses, a nice way to feel part of the process is to ask your child to paint the bump. Opt for safe, non-toxic paints such as facepaints that are intended for use on the skin. Be sure to take lots of photos of the process and the finished masterpiece.

Keep it real

Parents often try to change a toddler's routine when the new baby arrives. This can leave a toddler feeling pushed out, so try to introduce any changes a few months beforehand. This way your toddler is less likely to blame the new baby.

Keeping them in the loop

Make your child feel important. Encouraging them to be kind and helpful towards their younger sibling may empower them. You could ask for their help bathing the baby, to pass you nappies or to find a toy. However, always follow your child's lead. If they don't want to participate, that's fine. Just let them adjust to the new arrival in their own time.

Make a fuss of them

It is perfectly natural for any child to feel put out about the idea of a new baby stealing their thunder. If you approach the issue with a little sensitivity and some creativity, sibling rivalry is less likely to be an issue.

Sometimes when a new baby comes a toddler can feel left out with the array of cards and gifts brought for the baby. Have a word with guests and ask them to make a fuss of your toddler upon arrival. Make sure you remember to make a fuss of them too. You probably won't be up for running around a soft play centre, but while the baby is sleeping you could paint, colour, or have a cuddle watching their favourite DVD together.

Toddler troubles

Your toddler may become resentful towards the new baby. After all, he's had mum and dad all to himself for a long period of time, then all of a sudden he has to share them with a competitor. He may feel threatened, especially as a baby will take up so much of your time. It's a good idea to be aware of these feelings your toddler may have. They are very common and will ease as your children grow up. Even so, it's not advised to leave a baby alone with young children under 5: it is not uncommon for a toddler to pinch or even hit a baby. As mothers we can act like lionesses to protect our babies when they're threatened, even if the threat comes from another sibling! Try to remain calm, and gently explain that it's wrong to hurt people. Don't be tempted to smack your child as children tend to follow their parents' lead. If the situation continues, you could give your child a consequence, and if your child ignores your warning, enforce that consequence. It's important to always do so in a gentle way, however conflicted you may feel.

Sam: "When Yasmin was born I gave her a dolly from Ella. When I massaged Yasmin, Ella would copy my moves and massage her doll. We'd sing, talk and laugh. It was a great bonding experience for all of us."

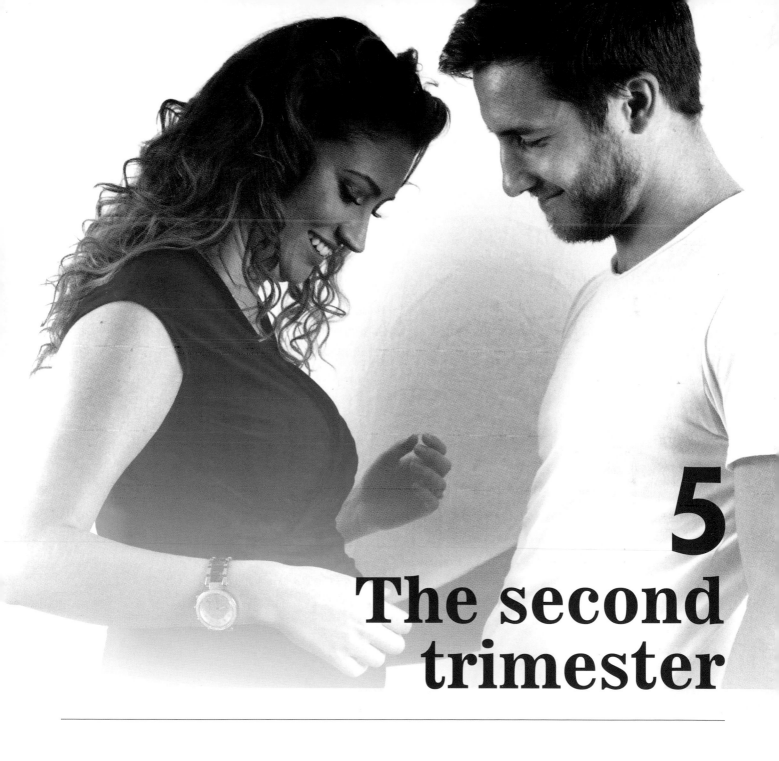

5
The second trimester

5
The second trimester

The second trimester is usually the most energetic. Morning sickness and fatigue have often subsided, and the baby is not so big as to cause problems with mobility or comfort. This is the point when many women really start to enjoy being pregnant.

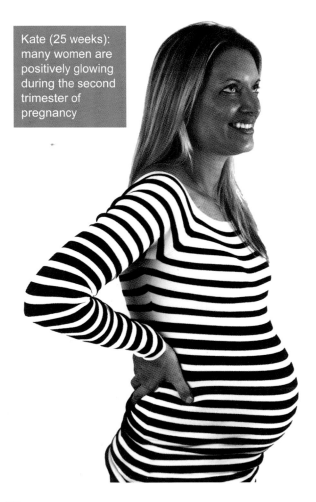

Kate (25 weeks): many women are positively glowing during the second trimester of pregnancy

Your state of mind

Your hormone imbalances are beginning to level out, and your moods will feel more stable. If you have kept the pregnancy quiet for the first trimester, you may find being able to tell people a huge relief, especially at work. Your body will need more rest. If you're so exhausted you can hardly stand, see if your boss will let you work from home one day a week, or when you really need it, or try some mindfulness at your desk. Please don't carry on regardless; you're growing another life inside you and you need to listen to your body.

At this stage, you might consider setting out your birthing plan, and coming up with a list of questions for your midwife, even if you don't make any definite decisions until the third trimester. Our active birth chapter is worth reading before you write your plan.

Your body

The most noticeable change will occur to your breasts. In the first trimester they would most likely have been rather tender and uncomfortable. In the second trimester, although less tender, they will continue to grow as they prepare for breastfeeding. You may notice that the skin

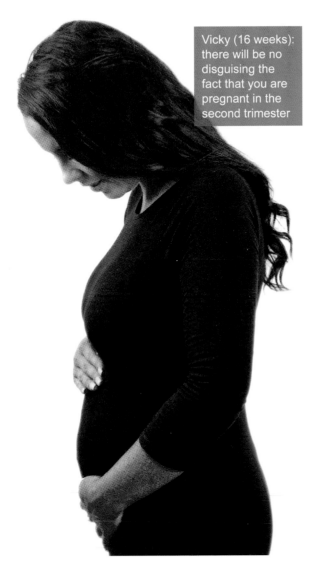

Vicky (16 weeks): there will be no disguising the fact that you are pregnant in the second trimester

Nutrient absorption is crucial in supporting your unborn baby,[1] and the process can lead to constipation and heartburn for you. You may find that you are sweating more because your metabolic rate has increased; the increase in blood volume boosts metabolism by about 20 per cent, creating more body heat.[2] You may also get a runny or stuffy nose or even the occasional nosebleed. This is due to your body going through hormonal changes, and your blood supply increasing. From week 17 onwards you are likely to put on around 1.3kg (3lb) a week in weight. Your ligaments will start to soften, so you will want to take care not to lift anything too heavy and to keep your body strong and flexible, perhaps using yoga.

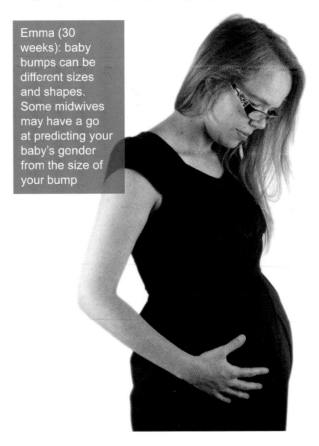

Emma (30 weeks): baby bumps can be different sizes and shapes. Some midwives may have a go at predicting your baby's gender from the size of your bump

around your nipples grows darker as the milk glands enlarge. There may even be a little leakage of colostrum (colostrum starts to form in your breasts during pregnancy; it contains antibodies to protect the newborn). All of this is your body's way of making sure you are ready to feed your baby when the time comes.

Pregnancy ailments

Here are some of the most common ailments, along with natural ways to treat them from home.

Backaches and pelvic aches

There is going to be a lot of strain on your back, pelvis and hips as your baby continues to grow. Pelvic pain is sometimes called pregnancy-related pelvic girdle pain (PPGP) or symphysis pubis dysfunction (SPD) and walking can feel uncomfortable.

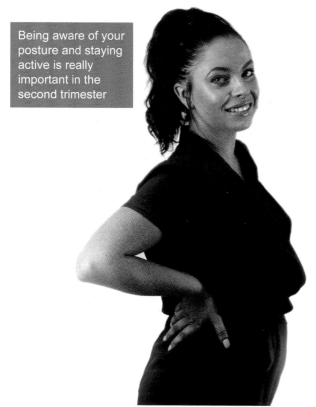

Being aware of your posture and staying active is really important in the second trimester

Posture pain

Many pregnant women walk with their baby bump pushed out in front of them, but this can strain their lower back muscles. Try to focus on your posture, try not to curve your spine and remember to stand tall. This will even help you to breathe more easily too.

Remedies

- **Massage**

Massage can soothe aching muscles and may be effective during labour as it triggers the body's natural pain relievers, endorphins.

Natural massage oil

½ cup of coconut oil
2 tbsp of sweet almond oil
5 drops of lavender essential oil
5 drops of mandarin oil
Glass jar or bottle

Melt ½ cup of coconut oil with 2 tbsp of sweet almond oil.

Add the drops of the essential lavender and mandarin oil

Pour the whole mixture into a clean jar or bottle and allow to cool.

Pop the cap on and use as a soothing massage oil whenever required.

- **Essential oils**

You should only use essential oils if you have no health concerns or complications. If you are at all unsure, consult your doctor.

When essential oils are inhaled or rubbed into the skin, they pass into the bloodstream and continue into the nervous system. Once there, they work on the limbic system, which is the part of the brain associated with emotions and the control of hormones. Modern scientists are now finding compelling links between scents and how it affects human behaviour.[3]

Each different oil has a slightly different effect on the limbic system. For example, lavender is great at reducing muscle pain and inflammation, as it is a natural antibiotic. It can also act as an antidepressant too.

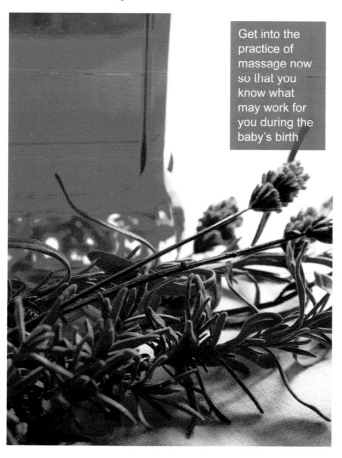

Get into the practice of massage now so that you know what may work for you during the baby's birth

Top tips for home massage

- Your birth partner should warm some carrier oil between their palms. Grapeseed oil is suitable for everyone

- Kneel in an upright position resting both of your shoulders against your bed. Put a pillow under your knees, and make sure there is no pressure on the bump. If you don't feel comfortable, reposition yourself

- Your birth partner should position their hands on your lower back either side of the spine (not the spine itself) and push their hands up your back until they reach the nape of your neck. Then return to the base of your spine, in light and wavy lines. Repeat this three times

- Next, rub both hands in a circular motion over your back and down into your waist

- Use the same motion over and around your buttocks, applying gentle pressure with the palms

- Use an unclenched fist to massage your neck, moving downwards to the hips on one side of the spine (this is great for relieving back pain). Next, move back up to the neck on the other side of the spine

- Repeat the first motion in long, soothing slow strokes.

Heartburn

Heartburn afflicts many women during pregnancy mainly due to the hormonal changes that your body is going through. Pregnancy hormones cause your muscles to relax; this includes the valve in your oesophagus (the tube that connects your mouth and stomach). If this valve doesn't close properly, then stomach acid can travel up it, which triggers a burning sensation.[4]

▪ Eat little and often

This is a good technique to bear in mind not just when it comes to heartburn, but if you want to reduce feelings of nausea and bloating. Eating small portions regularly throughout the day means that your stomach doesn't become too full and push your diaphragm up, which in turn sends that burning stomach acid to the oesophagus.

▪ Drink between meals

It is best to drink between meals rather than with them. Liquid dilutes the digestive juices, making them less effective at breaking down food, so digestion takes longer, which means there is more chance of heartburn.

▪ Probiotics

Probiotics leave friendly bacteria in the digestive system which aid digestion and lessen the chance of heartburn. You can buy probiotic supplements, but there are plenty of natural ways to obtain them too, including live yoghurts, sauerkraut, kefir and, rather wonderfully, dark chocolate (make sure it is at least 72 per cent cocoa solid).

▪ Ginger

Ginger in any form, including ginger ale and ginger biscuits, can soothe heartburn and nausea. You might like to make some homemade ginger tea using the recipe from the first trimester chapter.

▪ Herbal teas

Try peppermint or dandelion, or Mumma Love Organics' own recipe on the next page for heartburn tea, which is delicious, refreshing and soothing.

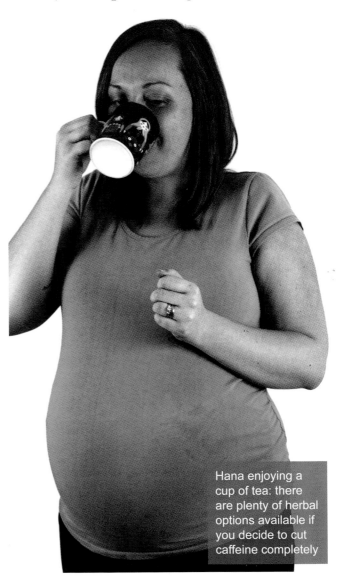

Hana enjoying a cup of tea: there are plenty of herbal options available if you decide to cut caffeine completely

Heartburn tea

The herbs in this tea have a calming anti-inflammatory effect on the digestive system, which will soothe reflux, heartburn and stomach upsets.

1 tbsp mint leaves
1 tsp fennel
1 tsp dill
1 cup of water

Remove stalks and chop each herb separately. Place in a saucepan and cover with water. Heat until warm but don't allow to boil – up to 80ºC (175ºF) is ideal.

Allow to infuse for 5 minutes before straining and serving.

■ Oats

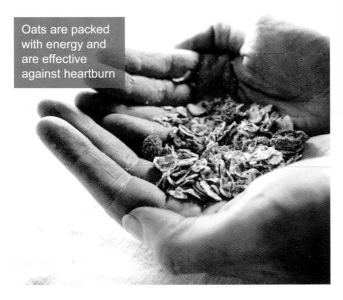

Oats are packed with energy and are effective against heartburn

Oats help to neutralize acidity levels, making them perfect for easing heartburn. The University of Maryland Medical Center says wholegrain foods are low in sugar and rich in B vitamins, effectively controlling acid reflux. Oatmeal is a great, inexpensive remedy for this problem.[5] Whether in porridge or muesli, oats are the ideal breakfast for pregnant women. They are also full of soluble fibre that will help to stabilize blood sugar levels. Try serving with dried fruit for extra iron and energy, seeds for omega-3s, a chopped banana for potassium, and berries for vitamin C.

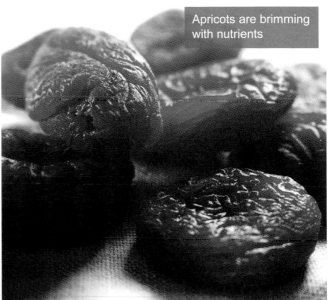

Apricots are brimming with nutrients

Anaemia

Anaemia occurs when there is a lack of oxygen-carrying red blood cells in the bloodstream.[6] In pregnancy it is essential that red blood cells increase, as they support the developing baby. Most cases of anaemia in pregnancy are due to a lack of iron, as red blood cells require iron to form. This is due to either diet, severe vomiting or rapid blood loss, for example during surgery.

Anything leafy and green (spinach, kale and watercress) is excellent at providing the iron needed to ensure adequate red-blood cell production. These vegetables are also high in folic acid.

To aid the absorption of iron into the body, iron-rich foods can be eaten with those that contain high amounts of vitamin C (including citrus fruits, strawberries, mangoes, tomatoes, cabbage, broccoli and peppers). Pomegranates are full of nutrients including iron, calcium and magnesium, and are rich in vitamin C. Apricots contain vitamin B complex, vitamin C and iron. A small portion of dried apricots is an ideal snack to carry around with you for a burst of energy between meals.

Constipation

Constipation is a common problem in pregnancy due to the pressure of the womb on the bowels. The good news is there are plenty of completely natural remedies.

■ High-fibre foods

The more fibre in your diet (whether you are pregnant or not), the better your undigested foods will move through the digestive tract, so that nothing becomes clogged up on the way. Getting your five to seven a day is more important than ever during pregnancy.

Raisins are excellent sources of fibre and natural laxatives, so a much better option than over-the-counter remedies that may cause problems for your developing baby.

Figs work in the same way as raisins, whether they are dried or fresh. Boiling some figs in milk and drinking this before bed is a brilliant way of staying regular.

Flaxseeds, almonds, fruits, and vegetables are packed full of fibre. If you don't always want to eat them, why not make them into a smoothie instead?

■ Hydration

Keeping hydrated during the day will stave off constipation. If you drink warm water first thing in the morning and last thing at night, it will help to stimulate the bowel, easing constipation.

■ Aromatherapy

Constipation can trigger painful cramps, but bathing in a warm bath with added lavender oil will help. Add four drops of lavender essential oil to a tablespoon of milk, before swirling it into your bath water. (The molecules in the oil will stick to the fat molecules in the milk and help them mix with the water, stopping them from evaporating.)

■ Exercise

Exercising, even gentle walking, offsets constipation by speeding up the time it takes the food to move through the intestines. It also accelerates breathing and your heart rate. This helps stimulate the natural flow of contractions to the intestinal muscles.

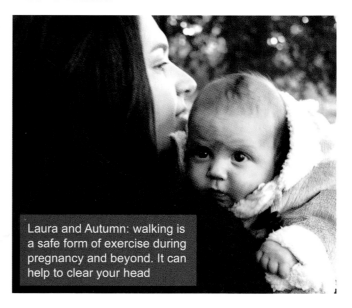

Laura and Autumn: walking is a safe form of exercise during pregnancy and beyond. It can help to clear your head

Yoga

Some yoga poses are ideal for combating constipation:

Easy pose

- Sit on the ground with your back straight

- Inhale and cross your legs. Exhale

- Sit up straight and place your hands on your knees or thighs

- Inhale and reach backwards with your arms straight and with your palms pressed together. Hold that position for four to six breaths

- Inhale and place one hand palm down on your back. Reach your other arm around your lower back and clasp your hands together while opening your chest. Hold for two breaths. Exhale

- Swap arms and repeat

- Inhale while reaching back with your arms straight. Clasp your hands together and hold for four to six breaths

- Inhale and place your palms on the floor behind you and lean back so that your abdomen, chest and back are open. Hold for two to four breaths

- Put your right hand on the floor behind your right thigh and inhale. Stretch your left arm up and lean to the right. Hold for two breaths. Repeat on the other side.

Modified seat twist

- Sit on the ground with your legs stretched out in front of you. Bend your right knee and place your right foot over your left knee. Place your left elbow over your right knee, while keeping your right hand on the floor for support

- Twist your body to the right and turn your head as far to the right as you can. Repeat on the opposite side.

Modified triangle pose

- Stand with your feet far apart in a triangle shape with your arms extended at shoulder level so that they are parallel with the floor

- Place your left hand straight over your head and bend down on your right-hand side to touch your right knee. Keep looking up at your left hand. Repeat on the other side.

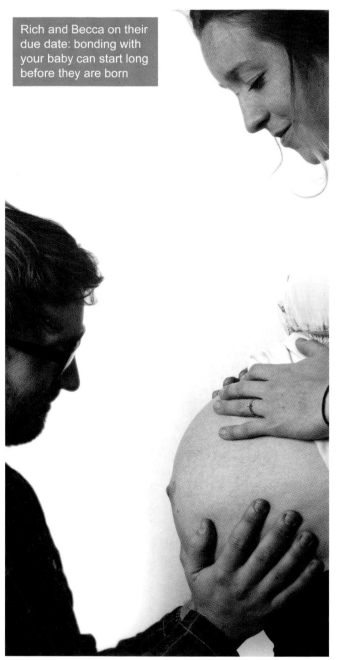

Stretchmarks

Stretchmarks are a very common part of pregnancy and are simply a change that our bodies may go through in order for us to have a beautiful baby. You can reduce stretchmarks by nourishing your skin and rubbing oils and creams (eg, the body butter recipe in the natural woman chapter) into your bump, which is also a lovely way to bond with your baby.

■ Coconut oil

Coconut oil has antiviral, antifungal, anti-inflammatory and antimicrobial properties. Coconut oil has incredible moisturizing powers, and the oil is quickly absorbed into the skin (it's also a great hair mask). It is an antioxidant so it fights the free radicals, which can damage the skin. Even better, topically applied coconut oil has no known side-effects.

■ Aloe vera gel

Aloe vera has many of excellent health-giving properties including the power to lessen stretchmarks and scarring. The gel can be bought processed, or you can make it yourself by squeezing it from the aloe vera plant. It is particularly effective if you have itchy dry skin.

■ Shea butter / cocoa butter

Just rub either of these directly on to the stretchmarks, and their appearance will, after continued use, be reduced. Shea butter will moisturize and improve the elasticity of your skin.

■ Keep hydrated

Getting enough water is essential for a healthy body and a healthy pregnancy. It also works to keep the skin supple and gives it greater elasticity, which means that stretchmarks are less likely.

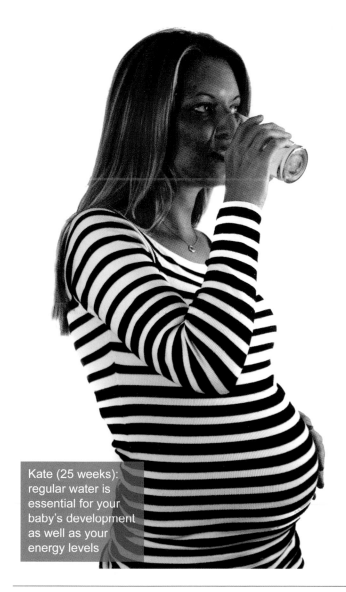

Kate (25 weeks): regular water is essential for your baby's development as well as your energy levels

■ Nutritious diet

Your skin needs nourishment too, so eat foods rich in vitamins C and E, silica and zinc, all of which are known to help clear and enrich the skin. Strawberries, blueberries, nuts, seeds, green beans, carrots, collard greens and spinach are just a few examples.

■ Vitamin E

Vitamin E is an antioxidant that protects the collagen fibres in your skin from damage by free radicals. Eat foods like spinach, olives, almonds, avocados and pumpkins, and rub vitamin E oil or cream into your skin as often as you think it is needed.

Sugar scrub

This is an easy home remedy that is great for reducing the appearance of stretchmarks and exfoliates the skin.

1 tbsp sugar
Lemon juice
Sweet almond oil
1 cup of water

Mix 1 tbsp of sugar with a few drops of lemon juice and a little sweet almond oil.

Mix together and apply.

Do this daily, and then take a warm bath.

Holly: "As time develops you'll be more aware of your baby's sleep cycles and can coordinate a light bump massage with when they are awake. If you do get stretchmarks, wear them proudly as a mark of your motherhood."

Sleeping positions

After the first trimester, it is best not to lie on your back for extended periods as this can affect the blood flow to the placenta and the baby. Lying on your back for 10-15 minutes at a time is fine, as long as you move if you start to feel light-headed.

In the second and third trimesters, sleeping on your left side is advised because this position will maximize blood flow to your baby. Left-sided sleeping during pregnancy prevents the uterus from applying pressure to the liver (which is on the right side of the body). It also improves blood flow to the foetus, the uterus and the kidneys and takes pressure off the back, which may alleviate typical pregnancy-related back pain.[7]

If you wake up and find that you have been sleeping on your back, don't worry. Your body will naturally reposition itself throughout the night. Your body knows what to do, have faith in it.

Things to do in the second trimester

Pick a birth partner

Most of the time it goes without saying that the father of the child will be present at the birth of your baby. However, this is not always possible. You could be preparing for pregnancy alone or your partner may work far away. If this is the case, your birthing partner could be a close friend, a family member, or even a doula. Decide on who would make you feel comfortable and empowered, and start the birthing conversation with them now.

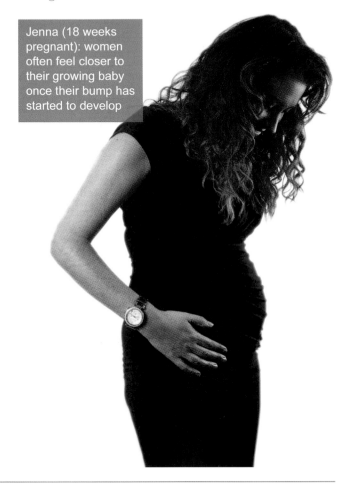

Jenna (18 weeks pregnant): women often feel closer to their growing baby once their bump has started to develop

---

Sam: "A doula provided the support I needed throughout the later stages of my second pregnancy and labour. I gave up cable TV to afford her service, and she was absolutely worth it."

Communicate with the bump

From 23 weeks, your baby's hearing will be well developed. Talk to the bump, so that they begin to recognize your voice. Try introducing your growing baby to different styles of music. Older siblings might enjoy talking to the bump too.

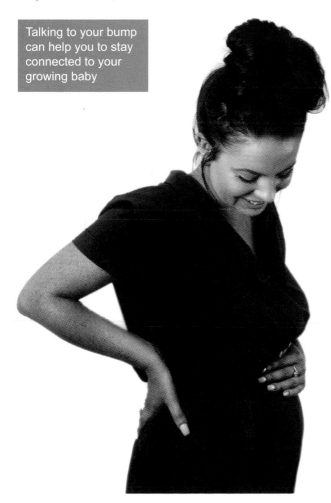

Talking to your bump can help you to stay connected to your growing baby

Mark the halfway point

Having a celebration halfway through the pregnancy can be really special. You are past the risky 12-week period, and without the lack of energy and discomfort that the third trimester can bring. You could celebrate with your partner, or close friends and family. You could ask everyone to bring a list of wishes for your baby to mount in a special book. Once the baby is born it can be hard to make the time to see people, so make the most of it while you can.

Stay fit

As well as doing the yoga exercises that help prevent constipation described earlier, you should keep working on the strength of your pelvic floor. In your second trimester you should continue practicing your Kegel exercises (p.63), if you haven't started those yet, by all means do start now! Having a strong pelvic floor will help you have more control of your bladder in the last stages of your pregnancy, and most importantly it will make it easier to push during your baby's birth. In the third trimester you might want to start massaging your perineum (p.94).

The developing baby – the second trimester[8]

Week 13
The placenta has taken over the maintenance of the pregnancy, and supplies the baby with oxygen and all the nutrients they need from their mother's diet. The baby's teeth have formed and lay in the gums.

Week 14

The baby responds to touch, and may move towards a hand placed on the mother's belly. Their limbs are fully formed and their kidneys are starting to function.

Week 15

The baby is growing rapidly and is able to move their head quickly. The braincells are multiplying at an astonishing rate. The baby weighs around 70g (2½oz) and could fit into the palm of your hand.

Week 16

Your baby is looking more human. At this point in the pregnancy, lanugo (fine hairs) are growing all over the body, and nerves are developing myelin sheaths, which speeds up the connections between body and brain.

Week 17

Your baby will be around 18cm (7") long and weigh about 140g (5oz). They will now be growing eyebrows and eyelashes!

Week 18

Breathing of a sort begins. The baby takes amniotic fluid into the lungs and breathes it back out in preparation for being born.

Week 19

The spinal cord is developing.

Week 20

At this stage, the baby is about half the length they will be when born. If they are is going to have hair at birth, this is when it begins to grow. The internal organs are now fully formed.

Week 21

The taste buds begin to develop.

Week 22

The baby will probably be able to differentiate between different voices and recognize certain sounds, such as favourite songs, as their ears are fully developed.

Week 23

Now those tiny hands are able to grip, and the limbs are almost completely developed.

Week 24

Your baby's eyes can open and close, and the lungs' air sacs are fully formed (although they would still have trouble breathing if born this early).

Week 25

You may sense when your baby is sleeping, as they will be establishing their own waking and sleeping patterns.

Week 26

Vernix now covers your baby. This is a greasy substance that waterproofs the new and delicate skin before birth.

Week 27

Another growth spurt will occur at around this stage, and there will be absolutely no missing the fact that you are pregnant!

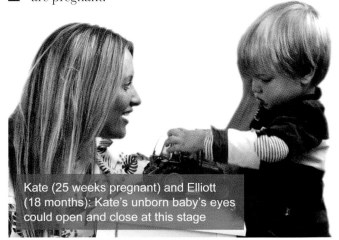

Kate (25 weeks pregnant) and Elliott (18 months): Kate's unborn baby's eyes could open and close at this stage

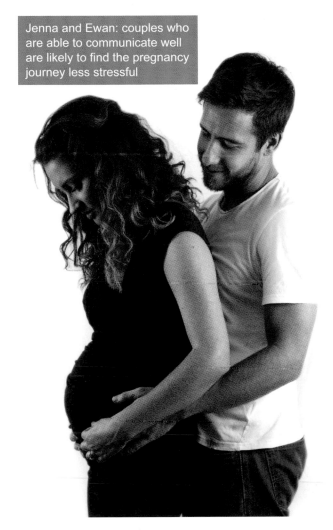

Jenna and Ewan: couples who are able to communicate well are likely to find the pregnancy journey less stressful

As your partner is likely to be more energetic and emotionally stable, this is a good time to organize everything that you'll need for your little one. You'll no doubt find that people will gift you a lot of clothing for your newborn, so don't invest too much at this stage. A safe sleeping space and a few key clothing items are essential, but it is a wise move to ignore the marketing cries that insist you splash out on all manner of fripperies. All a newborn really needs is your love, care and devotion.

You could think about what being a father means. It might be helpful to make a list of all the wonderful things that your father did for you. If you didn't have a great relationship with your father, consider all the things you'd like to do differently with your own child.

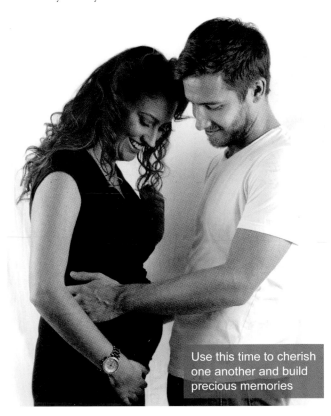

Use this time to cherish one another and build precious memories

Natural Dad

The pregnancy feels more real at this stage. Your partner will be obviously pregnant, so everyone will know about it. You'll find yourselves discussing practical matters, thinking about getting the baby's space in your house ready, and discussing the birth.

Writing a journal of insights, memories and your own experiences, including photos, could be a wonderful gift when they are older. No matter what happens, they will know that you were thinking about them before they were even born.

Journal for your child

Suggestions for your journal that will be a gift to your child:

- All the things I wish I'd known when I was a child

- My most important life lessons

- Things my father did that I am thankful for

- How I feel about being a father

- How I felt when I found out your mother was pregnant

- Things I want to change about the world

- Precious memories

- Life advice that everyone should know

- What we are doing to prepare for your birth

- Places I want to take you.

You could also add details of the pregnancy that feel significant to you.

Your partner may not feel quite with it for much of the pregnancy, so documenting the journey can be really worthwhile for all of you.

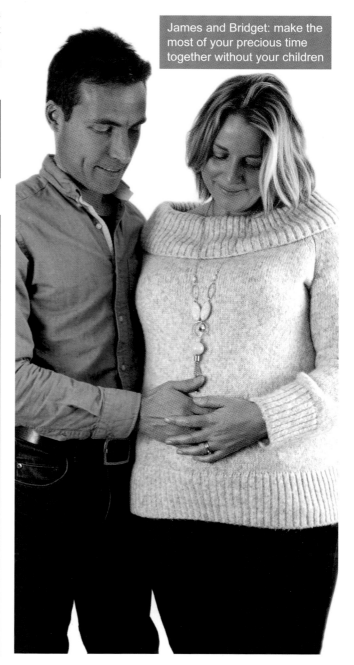

James and Bridget: make the most of your precious time together without your children

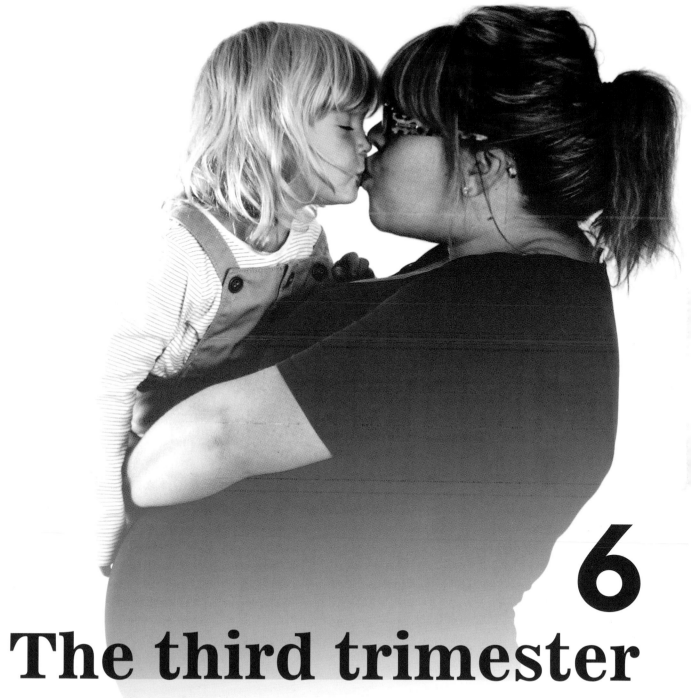

The third trimester

6

6
The third trimester

This is a really exciting time as there isn't long to wait before you'll get to meet your beautiful new baby! You may find that you are more tired than usual. You may feel uncomfortable as there is less room for your organs, the baby's weight is pushing on your bladder and pelvis, and sleep may be difficult. This is a good time to start focusing on life beyond the birth, and making sure that everything is in place for your little one's arrival.

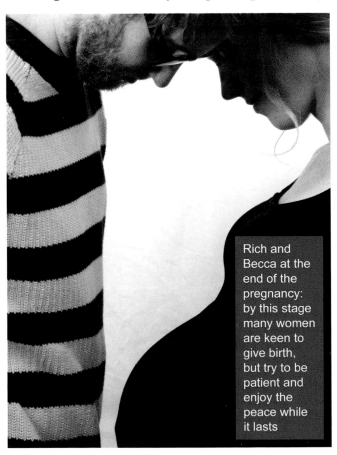

Rich and Becca at the end of the pregnancy: by this stage many women are keen to give birth, but try to be patient and enjoy the peace while it lasts

Your baby is getting bigger and stronger on a daily basis. Strong kicks and movements are hard to ignore, and it's worth keeping an eye on when your baby is usually most active so if there are any radical changes you can let your midwife or doctor know.

Stay healthy

It is really important that you keep up your nutritious diet, stay calm and relaxed, and drink plenty of water. Staying active can be difficult, especially in the last few weeks of pregnancy. You could take a gentle walk, or try some yoga stretches. If you feel remotely light-headed, simply stop what you are doing. It can help to lie with your legs up the wall and your body flat on the floor, bringing the blood back to your head. Breathe deeply in this position. To ease the hip ligaments you could bend the knees outwards like frog's legs, pushing your knees towards the wall.

Fluid retention

Around 50 per cent of all pregnant women experience fluid retention / oedema, especially in the third trimester. Your feet, ankles and calves may swell, especially if you are on your feet a lot. Try to rest whenever possible and keep your feet elevated above your hips.

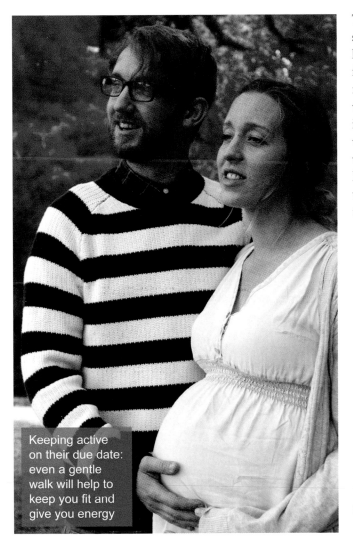

Keeping active on their due date: even a gentle walk will help to keep you fit and give you energy

To help your body flush out the excess fluid, you need to support your kidneys. A clean, healthy diet will give your kidneys less to filter, so avoid processed sugar, saturated fats and salt. Salt is especially bad for exacerbating fluid retention. It is also vital that you keep drinking plenty of water. Many fruit and vegetables have a high water content, including cabbage and watercress (natural diuretics which will help to reduce excess fluid in your body), salad vegetables, asparagus, carrots, grapes and watermelon. During the summer months, you can freeze cubes of watermelon and even whole grapes for a refreshing snack that will help to hydrate you.

Natural diuretic

Combining natural diuretics will fight fluid retention, and top up your vitamins and minerals.

In a blender, whizz up:

2 handfuls of fresh parsley

4 sticks of celery

2 apples (cored)

1 glass of cranberry juice

Holly: "I kept physically active while I was carrying Jasmine by walking, swimming and regular yoga practice. Towards the end of the third trimester I was able to manage much less, but the regular exercise I did earlier in the pregnancy helped to give me the stamina I needed for an active birth."

Dandelion leaves have a gentle diuretic effect and are also high in potassium, which can help if fluid retention is caused by high sodium levels in the body. (Bananas are another great source of potassium.) If you don't feel up to traipsing about your local park looking for dandelions, you could instead find this grassy-tasting tea in many healthfood stores. You can always add a squeeze of fresh lemon juice to make the tea more palatable.

Dandelion leaf tea

Dandelion leaves are very rich in iron and vitamin K and have diuretic qualities. You can nibble on them as a snack, or add them to salads.

If you happen to have an abundance of dandelions growing nearby, or a spirited toddler who might like to join you on a dandelion-picking mission, try your hand at making your own tea:

Pick the young tender leaves as close to the root as possible. You only need a handful for a cup of tea.

Wash them thoroughly before roughly chopping them.

Add them to a mug, then pour in boiling water and leave them for 10 minutes. (If you leave them too long, they will start to taste bitter.)

You could combine the tea with organic apple juice, or chill the tea and combine it with plenty of water, ice cubes and lemon slices.

Calf massage

A calf massage will help to drain fluid from the calves, ankles and feet. You could use a good carrier such as grapeseed oil, or you may prefer to mix up an aromatherapy blend of essential oils with diuretic effects:

Add
3 drops of grapefruit oil
2 drops of geranium oil
1 drop of lavender oil
to 15ml (½fl oz) carrier oil

Sit in a chair with your massage buddy cross-legged on the floor before you. After warming the oil in their palms, they should massage from your ankle to your knee in small circles. Let them know if the pressure is too much as the swelling may be uncomfortable. After the massage, leave your feet elevated above hip height for a good half an hour.

Alternatively, add the essential oils (without the carrier oil) to a large bowl of warm water and submerge your feet and ankles for 5 minutes. It is worth combining the essential oils with a dash of milk to stop them from evaporating.

Sam: "I love how aromatherapy can lift your mood, as well as treat physical ailments. I found that grapefruit was uplifting and restored my sense of well-being, geranium helped to make me feel calm, and lavender was so relaxing."

Sam: "Nothing beats the feeling of connection you get when massaging your bump, especially when your baby responds to your movements."

Pre-eclampsia

Although this serious condition can develop from 20 weeks onwards, it is most common in the third trimester. Pre-eclampsia occurs when the placenta isn't working as it should be.

If you have swelling in your legs and ankles that leave an indention when pressed, or you suddenly get dramatic swelling in your hands, face or feet, this could be a sign of pre-eclampsia. Other symptoms include problems with your vision, severe headaches, and pain below the ribcage. It is vital that you call your midwife if you notice any of these symptoms. Early signs include high blood pressure and protein in your urine. Mild pre-eclampsia affects up to 6 per cent of pregnancies, and severe cases develop in about 1-2 per cent of pregnancies. There is nothing to stop you going on to have a healthy baby, but you will need medical attention.[1]

Connect with your baby

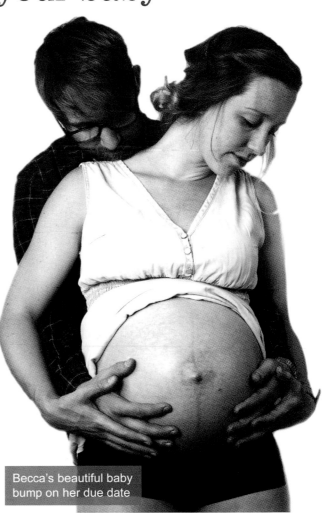

Becca's beautiful baby bump on her due date

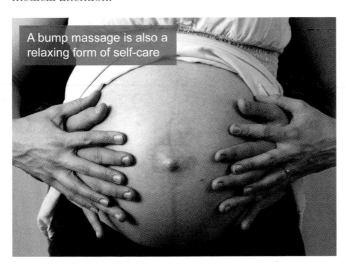

A bump massage is also a relaxing form of self-care

Bump massage

½ cup of coconut oil
2 tbsp of sweet almond oil
5 drops of lavender essential oil
5 drops of mandarin oil
Glass jar or bottle

Melt ½ cup of coconut oil with 2 tbsp of sweet almond oil.

Add the drops of the essential lavender and mandarin oil

Pour the whole mixture into a clean jar or bottle and allow to cool.

Pop the cap on and use as a soothing massage oil whenever required.

Exercising for labour

The healthier your body is, the easier you'll find labour. You may struggle to stay active during the third trimester, so you might like to try these exercises instead.

Supported squats

Active birth positions (where the mother is encouraged to move around and find the positions that suit her best) rely on gravity, so having strong legs can be really helpful.

- With your legs a hip-width apart, hold on to the back of the chair that someone is sitting on (for ballast), a mantelpiece or a solid surface

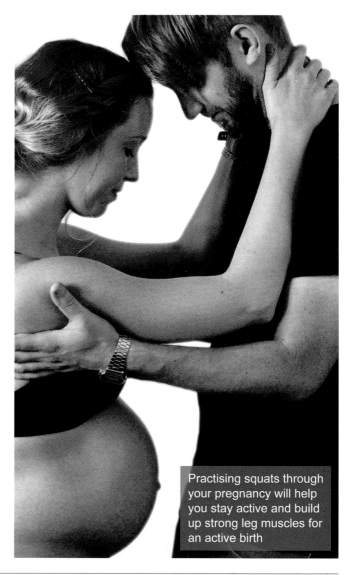

Practising squats through your pregnancy will help you stay active and build up strong leg muscles for an active birth

Holly: "Trying out various active birth positions helped me to have a faster and uncomplicated labour, and all the pregnancy yoga, walking and swimming meant I was able to stay upright throughout the birthing process."

- Keeping a straight back, slowly squat until your thighs are parallel to the ground
- Hold for a few seconds and stand
- Try to co-ordinate the movement with your breath, breathing out as you squat and inhaling as you return to standing
- Keep the movements slow and controlled
- Try to do up to two sets of fifteen a day for the final trimester of your pregnancy. Stop immediately if you feel light-headed or breathless.

Swimming

Swimming can build stamina in preparation for labour as well as keeping limbs strong. It can be a break for women who feel weighed down by their bump and appreciate the support from the water. Water also takes the pressure off the pelvis.

Using a birthing ball

A birthing ball will help you to maintain core strength throughout your pregnancy. As long as your hips are higher than your knees, a birthing ball can be surprisingly comfortable. (It's basically the same as an exercise ball, but a birthing ball may cost more.) Investing in one now means that you can strengthen your core during the postnatal period and also use it during labour, to help ease contractions.

Sit on your birthing ball throughout the day and your muscles will do the work for you. Rotate your hips in a figure of eight: this can encourage the baby to drop down into the pelvis in preparation for birth. Alternatively, lean your upper body on the exercise ball for support and rotate your hips in a figure of eight to help your baby move into position and relieve some of the pressure on your pelvis during the last few weeks of pregnancy.

Pelvic tilts

To keep your lower back supple and your pelvis mobile, rest on all fours and curl your tailbone under as you breathe in and release it as you breathe out. This movement can also ease lower back pain. If your baby is in a posterior position, this gentle rocking motion can encourage them to move into an anterior position (ideal for birth). Wait until the baby is active, and try some slow, rhythmical pelvic tilts to encourage the baby to settle into a better birthing position. Try the pelvic tilt three times a day, for no more than five minutes at a time.

Seated frog legs

Sit on a cushion or pillow with your knees together and your feet flat on the floor. Stretch your spine up towards the ceiling and inhale deeply. As you exhale let your knees drop out to the sides and bring the soles of your feet together. Lean forwards gently, and use your elbows to push down on the knees to create a gentle stretch. This posture will stretch the legs and keep the pelvis open and loose, as well as taking the pressure off the lower back. Try holding the pose for five seconds and doing five repetitions.

Nutrition

It is really essential that your diet is rich in iron. Not only because your blood is playing such a vital role in the development of your baby and the placenta, but also because there is some blood lost during labour and in the weeks following the birth (lochia).[2]

As well as iron, your body will need plenty of calcium. During the seventh and eighth months of pregnancy your baby's cartilage will turn into bone. They will use your calcium stores to get what they need, so it is especially important to include plenty of calcium in your diet.

Your baby's brain is growing faster than ever, so keeping yourself topped up with omega-3s is another crucial element of your diet, with two servings of fish a week, although avoid those with a high mercury content (like shark, swordfish, king mackerel and tilefish).[3] Our bodies do not produce omega-3s so your baby will rely on your diet to get the omega-3s required. In the USA for example, most Americans' diets are seriously lacking in omega-3 fats. Studies show that adequate omega-3 intake during pregnancy, breastfeeding, infancy and beyond has a positive impact on the intelligence of the child.[4]

Braxton Hicks

Braxton Hicks contractions are a very common and healthy part of pregnancy. They occur throughout pregnancy (from around six weeks) but we often don't feel them until the third trimester, and many women don't feel them at all. They tend to be irregular and can be uncomfortable. They have a similar squeezing tightening sensation to real contractions but for the majority of women they are painless.

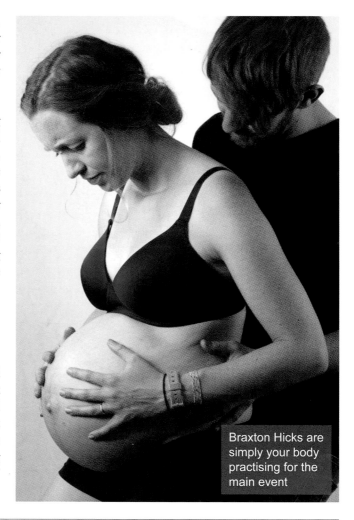

Braxton Hicks are simply your body practising for the main event

Sam: "It can be tricky to decipher between Braxton Hicks and real contractions, especially the first time round. Stay calm, practise your deep breathing and make a note of how long each contraction lasts and how regularly it comes. If you are in any doubt, then ring your midwife or maternity unit if you are giving birth in hospital."

During the last few weeks or days of pregnancy, Braxton Hicks contractions can become more rhythmical and close together. This is known as false labour. In actual labour the contractions will become more frequent and stronger.

If you find that your Braxton Hicks contractions are getting a bit uncomfortable, then you might find a relaxing bath soothing. Otherwise, use your deep breathing and mindfulness exercises to relax. These exercises are also useful in the early stages of labour.

Unless your doctor has informed you otherwise, it is usual not to contact the midwife or hospital until you've had an hour of regular contractions that come every 5 minutes and last around 60 seconds each time. Make sure you have a watch or a clock with a second hand. It can be quite hard to time your own contractions so ideally your birth partner will have a suitable watch too.

Nesting

Nesting instincts are very common during the last few weeks of the third trimester. Don't try to fight this feeling; it is perfectly natural and going with your instincts will help you to feel more prepared for the baby's arrival.

Stretchy feelings in the abdomen

Feeling as if your abdomen is being pulled is perfectly normal during the later stages of pregnancy. Keep the skin well nourished, or use our bump massage to soothe yourself as well as bond with the baby.

Rest and sleep

Many women struggle to sleep during the later part of pregnancy; this may be due to frequent urination, discomfort or persistent worries. Get in the habit of free writing before bed so that your mind isn't dwelling on troublesome thoughts. It can also help to write a to-do list for the next day. If you lie in bed and start to think about what needs to be done, it can really disturb your sleep. You may like to practise some mindfulness and relax with a soothing bump massage. Establishing a good sleep routine for yourself now will help you once the baby is born.

If you aren't getting enough sleep at night, then it is imperative that you sleep during the day. Giving birth will demand all your energy, whether you opt for a c-section, have an assisted delivery or give birth naturally.

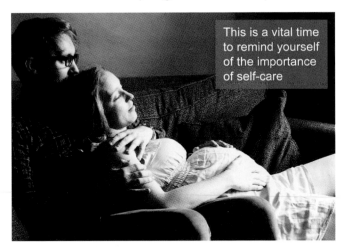

This is a vital time to remind yourself of the importance of self-care

Sit on the floor

Try to get in the habit of sitting on the floor as much as possible. You can use a cushion if it makes you more comfortable. It will improve your posture, help to keep your core strong and prepare your body for an active birth.

Too much time spent in an armchair or on a sofa can cause slouching; without the support of a chair we have to engage the muscles in our back and abs to remain upright, so this is a great way to strengthen the core without too much exertion.

A cross-legged position is great for strengthening the leg muscles and opening the pelvis.

Vaginal stretching and perineal massage

Both these exercises are recommended only after the 34th week. The vagina is perfectly designed to stretch and contract, but keeping these muscles pliable and flexible reduces the risk of tearing.

Position yourself on the floor with your legs wide apart. Insert both index fingers into the vagina and pull down towards your anus for 30 seconds before releasing. Work all around the vagina in this manner, breathing deeply and visualizing your vagina opening up. It can be helpful to imagine it gently expanding like a bud and blossoming into a flower. And when you go into labour, this visualization will help you to relax the area.

Preparing the perineum, by keeping the tight muscles between the vagina and anus flexible, will also help your body open up easily. Stretch those muscles every day: rub in a circular motion using your fingertips and organic olive oil – perhaps after a bath or shower, when the muscles are already relaxed.

It may feel a little strange to massage your perineum or practice vaginal stretching, but these exercises not only keep

the area pliable and flexible – they also keep you connected with your body. This is the perfect time to use the vagina to its full potential. After the birth you'll have a whole new kind of respect for your amazing sex organs.

Raspberry leaf tea

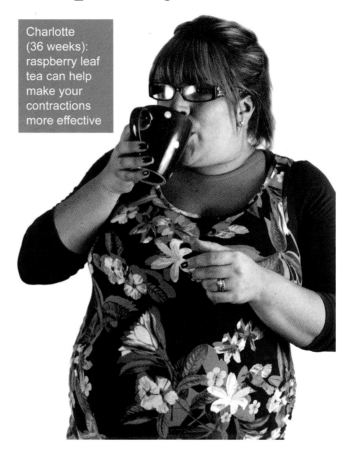

Charlotte (36 weeks): raspberry leaf tea can help make your contractions more effective

This uterine tonic, available from supermarkets and most healthfood stores, will help strengthen the uterus, making contractions more powerful and helping you to give birth at a nice steady pace. There is some evidence to suggest that raspberry leaf tea may help to prevent the need for a c-section or assisted delivery.[5] It can also help to protect against postnatal haemorrhage. You can drink one cup a day from 24 weeks onwards. Try drinking 2 cups a day from 30 weeks, building up to 3 cups from 36-37 weeks. If you don't enjoy the taste, sweeten with honey. It is advisable to slowly build up the doses in this manner, as your pregnancy develops. If you suddenly start drinking a lot of raspberry leaf tea when you are overdue, it may cause contractions that are so intense that your baby becomes distressed.[6]

Sex

As long as there are no complications, it is perfectly fine to make love during the whole of your pregnancy. Sperm is a natural source of prostaglandins,[7] which is used synthetically to induce labour. This doesn't mean that sex can cause premature labour, rather that it can encourage things along when you are nearing your due date. So if things aren't progressing as quickly as you'd like, sex might be the answer to gently put the wheels in motion!

Bonding

By week 31, your baby will be able to differentiate between light and dark[8] and taste the foods that you eat. So that light isn't such a shock when they come into the world, expose the bump to light where possible, ideally when the baby is awake and active. Pregnant women are more sensitive to the sun's rays, so always protect your skin before exposing it to sunlight.

Maintaining a varied diet will mean that your baby is introduced to a variety of different tastes. If you plan on breastfeeding, be aware that certain strong flavours can come through in the milk. Most of our food preferences are learned, and a growing body of research shows that this learning also begins before birth. By introducing

your baby to a variety of different tastes now, you may be able to continue this through the breastfeeding and weaning period.[9]

You might like to play soothing music to the bump. If your unborn associates that music with a feeling of serenity, you may be able to use the same music to soothe them to sleep or to help keep them calm once they are born. Amniotic fluid is a good conductor of sound, so play music at a level that feels comfortable to you. Your baby can also identify your voice, so speaking to them now may mean they are soothed by your voice after the birth.[10]

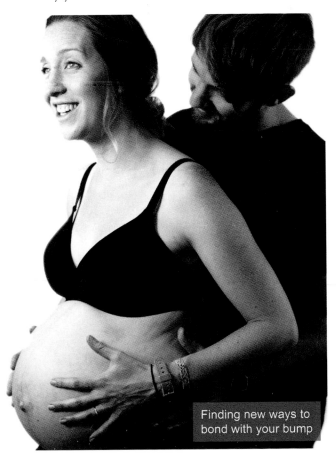

Finding new ways to bond with your bump

Realistic expectations

Although this book is focused on preparing your body for an active birth, whereby you are free to move around during labour to find positions that work best for you, it is also important to prepare yourself in case you are not able to do things naturally. Staying physically active and strong, keeping in touch with your body, bonding with your unborn baby and looking after yourself can all help you to give birth naturally. However, complications can occur with any birth and having a child by caesarean section or assisted delivery is a possibility for everyone.

When it comes to writing your birth plan, consider all the options should your ideal birth scenario become overridden by events.

Sleeping positions

As with the second trimester, you'll want to avoid sleeping on your back as this can restrict blood flow to the baby and the placenta. Ideally, you'll keep sleeping on your left-hand side so that more blood and nutrients will flow to the baby and the placenta.

You may find it harder to get comfy as your bump grows much bigger. It can help to place a pillow beneath the bump to support yourself during the night, which will also take some of the strain off your lower back. Placing a pillow between your knees will keep your hips aligned and will take pressure off the pelvis.

If you are getting up to wee more frequently in the night, having to reposition pillows every time that you settle down to sleep may seem a bit of a hassle. However, as your ligaments soften and the baby increases in weight, it is really important that you protect your back and pelvis.

Things to do in the third trimester

Refine your birth plan (and read up on the stages of birth)

Read up about different types of birth, talk to people about their own experiences and talk openly with your partner or birth partner. Having a detailed birth plan in place will help you to feel more in control.

Holly: "Ultimately, all we really want is a healthy baby. If you need a caesarean, focus on the positivity of getting to meet your child sooner and find ways to ensure that you still feel in control of the process. This might involve you choosing music or asking if you can use a mirror to observe the procedure. Having a specific birthing appointment time means you can plan exactly what happens before the birth."

Sam: "I wish I'd taken more opportunities to rest the first time round. I had no idea how exhausting caring for a newborn can be. I can't stress enough just how important it is to get as much sleep as possible during pregnancy."

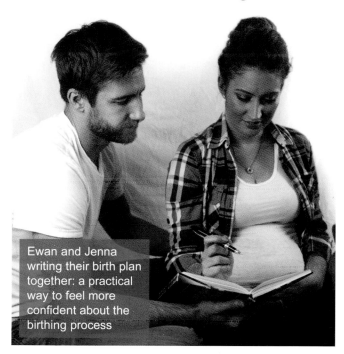

Ewan and Jenna writing their birth plan together: a practical way to feel more confident about the birthing process

Construct your baby equipment and prepare their room

The last thing that you'll feel like doing with a newborn is building furniture and constructing prams. Many women feel a slump in energy during the final weeks, so get everything ready while you are feeling energetic and rested. If you are tired, refer to your list of friends and family and ask someone practical to give you a hand.

Take some photos of your bump

You will no doubt find yourself taking many pictures of your new baby, but many women forget to take bump pictures before the big day arrives. Ask an artistic friend to take pictures of your pregnant self and your partner. These will be a lovely memory that you can show your little one when they are older.

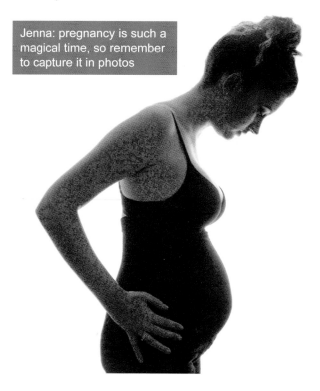

Jenna: pregnancy is such a magical time, so remember to capture it in photos

Bulk-cook healthy meals

When your baby is born, you will want to focus on their needs: feeding them, bathing them, helping them ease into a sleep routine and simply spending time together. You may not have the time or energy to cook, but your body will still need nutritious meals in order to heal after the birth.

Stews, soups, pies, tagines, curries, casseroles, homemade pizzas, moussaka and crumbles all freeze well. Make sure that these meals are packed with plenty of fresh vegetables to keep your energy levels high. Spend a day bulk-cooking a number of tasty recipes and freeze them all, labelling them clearly with the date they were made and what they are. These may also be helpful if you spend time in hospital and your partner hasn't the time to cook. There are plenty of nutritious recipes available on our website with advice on freezing, if you need any inspiration.

Read up about newborns and breastfeeding

With the day that you finally get to meet your baby being only weeks (or maybe days) away, this is the perfect time to learn more about how to care for a newborn and to think about breastfeeding. Focusing on the wonderful aspects of becoming a new parent may be helpful, especially if you are nervous about the birth itself.

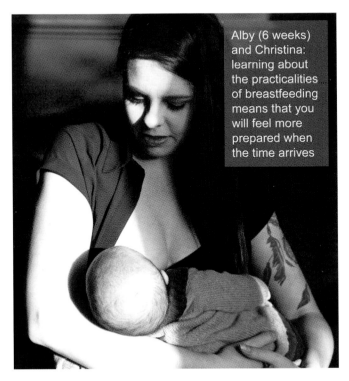

Alby (6 weeks) and Christina: learning about the practicalities of breastfeeding means that you will feel more prepared when the time arrives

The developing baby – the third trimester[11]

Week 28
Your baby's eyes are partially open and their eyelashes are formed. Your baby will be gaining in weight and their skin will be losing its many wrinkles.

Holly: "I made sure that I read everything that I could get my hands on so I was fully armed with all the facts long before Jasmine was born. Trying to get my head around all that after the birth would have been overwhelming."

Week 29

Your baby will be able to completely open their eyes and will probably have a full head of hair. Now that the bones are developed, red blood cells are forming within the bone marrow.

Week 30

The development of the central nervous system continues. Your baby will even be able to control their own body temperature.

Week 31

Your baby will start to shed its lanugo (the soft downy hair that has been covering their body) and will start to absorb vital vitamins and minerals from the intestinal tract. The tiny toenails are formed at this stage too. Your baby's lungs still have a bit of a way to go, but that won't stop them from inhaling and exhaling fluids to prepare them for breathing. They get all the oxygen they need from the umbilical cord.

Week 32

Your baby can not only detect light, but their pupils can also dilate at this stage. Your baby's skull will still be quite pliable, ready for the birth. The bones of the body will be harder too. As the fat builds up beneath your baby's skin they will become less red and wrinkly.

Week 33

Your baby's fingernails will have grown to the tips of their fingers. Their hearing will be fully developed. It is thought that babies respond to high-pitched tones. Your baby's lungs are almost fully developed at this stage, although the central nervous system is still growing.

Week 34

Your baby should gain around 225g (½lb) a week from now on. You may find that your baby has distinct waking and sleeping cycles now, as the womb stretches, enabling more light to filter through. Your baby's kidneys are fully developed and their liver is able to process a small amount of waste. Babies wee in the womb, adding to the amniotic fluid.

Week 35

Your baby will have less room to move as by now they are filling most of the amniotic sac. The head may also engage, giving your lungs and stomach a little more room. By the beginning of week 37 your baby will be full-term. You could give birth any day.

Week 36

Now that your baby is full-term, their organs can function alone. With your baby's head in your pelvic cavity, they have space to stretch their growing legs. Your baby will have swallowed all of the secretions and waste products, including the lanugo and some of the vernix caseosa (the white substance that covers the lanugo). This will be stored in their bowels until after the birth, when they will be released in the meconium (sticky black early poos).

After 37 weeks

Your baby's brain will continue to grow and their lungs will be the last thing to develop. It is common for babies to be born a week or two before or after their due date.

Hospital-bag essentials

Even if you are planning on a home birth, it can be handy to pack a hospital bag in case. The last thing you want to think about in labour is what to take to hospital with you!

It might be advisable to pack two bags, one for the labour and the other for the hospital stay. You will want to have everything ready from 36 weeks onwards. Check with the hospital first in case they have any restrictions on what you can bring with you. Some hospitals will limit pillows and birthing balls due to lack of space.

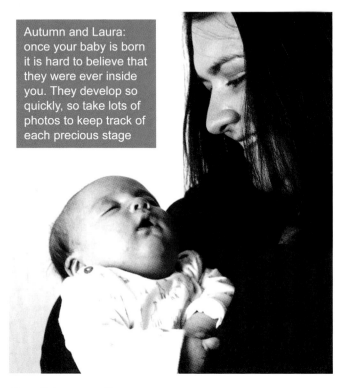

Autumn and Laura: once your baby is born it is hard to believe that they were ever inside you. They develop so quickly, so take lots of photos to keep track of each precious stage

Labour bag

- Your birth plan and notes
- A lightweight dressing gown
- An oversized T-shirt or nightshirt
- Warm socks (ideally with gripped soles)
- Drinks and snacks – for yourself and your birth partner (water, fruit juice, dried fruit, nuts and seeds are ideal)
- Massage oil
- Essential oils (used in massage and inhalations as an effective form of pain relief)

- Lip-balm (many women complain of dry lips in hospital)
- Water mist (a light facial mist can be very refreshing and cooling)
- Hair bands and grips (to keep your hair from your face)
- A birthing ball and pump (it is easier for your birthing partner to inflate it in the hospital than trying to negotiate you and a fully inflated birthing ball from the car park to the maternity unit, especially if you need a wheelchair)
- Things to do (if the labour is slow to progress then you might want to have a book to read or something to keep you occupied)
- A TENS (transcutaneous eletrical nerve stimulation) machine
- Music (making a birthing playlist is a lovely thing to do during the third trimester)
- A stress toy (something to squeeze to save your birth partner's hand!).

These are just suggestions. A TENS machine can restrict movement but may be very useful in the early stages of labour. Music can create a fantastic atmosphere, though some women find that they can't cope with music or even voices during labour. It is worth having as many options as possible available, as you won't know how you will feel until the time comes.

Post partum hospital bag

- Snacks and drinks (again keep it nutritious and healthy, with a little chocolate as a treat)
- A couple of clean nightdresses
- Maternity pads
- Toiletries
- A going home outfit (your womb will still be swollen so opt for something roomy and comfy)
- Nursing bras

- Big knickers
- Make-up (the last thing that some women feel like doing is putting on make-up, but others will feel more confident around visitors and in photos with some warpaint to hand)
- A list of phone numbers or a mobile and charger
- Lavender essential oil (great for promoting sleep and for healing).

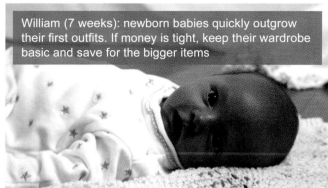

William (7 weeks): newborn babies quickly outgrow their first outfits. If money is tight, keep their wardrobe basic and save for the bigger items

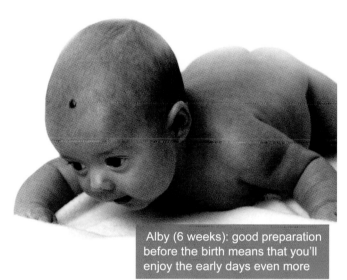

Alby (6 weeks): good preparation before the birth means that you'll enjoy the early days even more

For baby

- Sleepsuits and vests (pack plenty)
- Nappies (a newborn can get through 12 a day)
- A blanket (for leaving hospital and for photos)
- Muslin squares
- Hats, socks and booties
- Maybe even a cuddly toy (knowing that a particular toy has been with them since the day they were born could mean a lot to your child in the future).

You will also need a car seat for getting home (worth leaving in the car that is going to drive you to the hospital).

You may also want particular items that make you feel comforted and secure to hand. This could be photos of the family, a drawing from an older child, a treasured item from a grandparent or even a favourite scent.

Natural Dad

You are likely to find that your partner is able to do less during her final trimester. This may mean that you are looking after older children, doing the lion's share of the housework and taking care of your partner more than usual. This might be a good time to review the self-care chapter in this book. You need to be sure that you are well rested before the baby arrives so that you can support your partner through the birth and through the postnatal period.

Keep eating a balanced diet and stay hydrated. Exercise might prove helpful at this point, especially if you feel overwhelmed by responsibility. Keep yourself as healthy as possible, and you'll be in the best position to look after your family.

Talk to your partner about what they expect from you and how you'll best be able to help. Understanding each stage of labour means that you'll be able to better support your partner, so arm yourself with as much knowledge as possible.

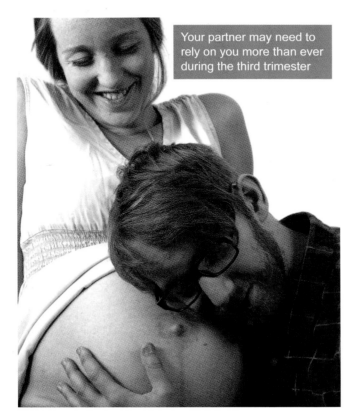

Your partner may need to rely on you more than ever during the third trimester

Don't forget to pack your own hospital bag in advance too. You might like to include a change of clothes, drinks, snacks, your camera, basic toiletries, a book, and enough change for the hospital car park.

Writing a birth plan together will help you to understand what your partner wants from the birth. Knowing what her expectations are means that you will be there to support her and to communicate her wishes to the midwife or birthing team. You may find that during labour she finds it difficult to have a conversation with you, so staying in tune with her needs before labour should help. You may need to request gas and air, for example, if she is busy fielding contractions.

You might need to make a plan of what to do if your partner goes into labour while you are working. Is there a friend who can be with your partner until you arrive? How are you going to get to the hospital?

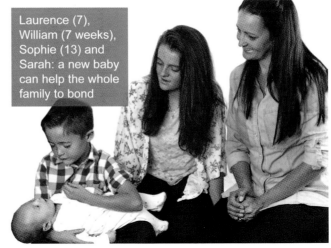

Laurence (7), William (7 weeks), Sophie (13) and Sarah: a new baby can help the whole family to bond

Danny, father to Eloise (3 months): "When my wife was around 7 months pregnant I felt so anxious. I tried to keep it from her, but it only caused distance between us. When we eventually spoke about my worries, I realized that she felt a similar way. Ultimately, it deepened our relationship and made me realize that I didn't need to be strong for her, but we could feel fragile together."

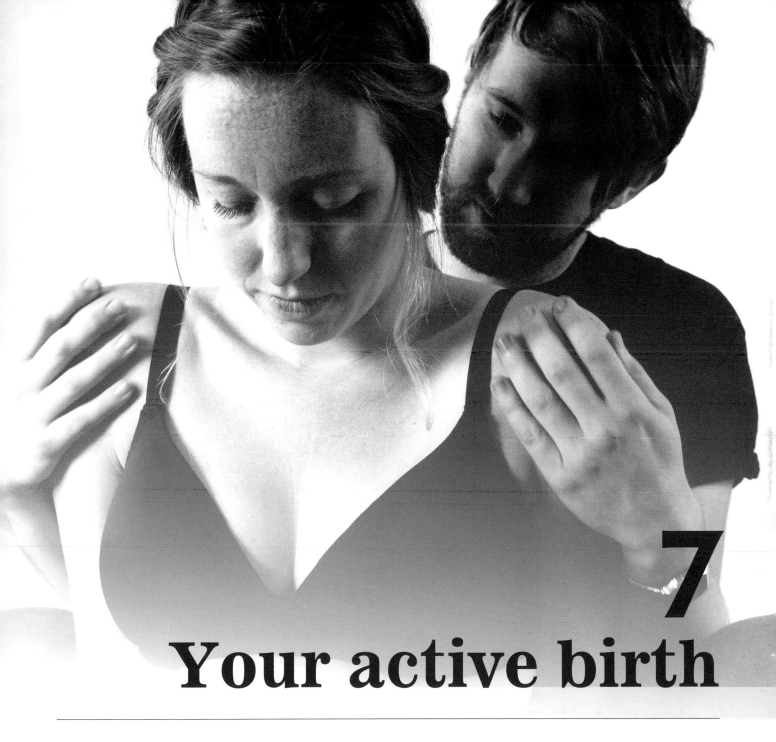

Your active birth

7

7
Your active birth

With our wide pelvises and the miracle of an expandable cervix and vagina, we women are built to give birth. Our bodies know exactly what to do, we just need to tap into our instinct. This may sound like a straightforward concept but in practice it can seem a little overwhelming.

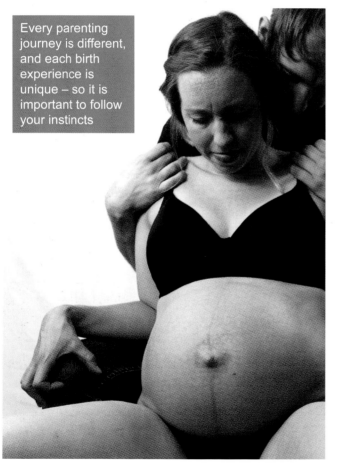

Every parenting journey is different, and each birth experience is unique – so it is important to follow your instincts

During pregnancy you may feel as though the body you once thought you knew well is no longer yours, so before the birth is the ideal time to try to connect with yourself.

If you have been practising mindfulness and yoga throughout your pregnancy, feeding your body with nutritious meals and dealing with ailments in a natural way, then you will be in an ideal place to listen to your body's cues. Even if you haven't, there is still plenty you can do to help tune in to your instinct.

Know what to expect

Many women are terrified by the idea of giving birth. This could be because of a negative birth experience in the past or sensational media portrayal. If someone starts to pour out their dramatic birthing story to you, it is perfectly ok to remind them that it may not be the best time for you to hear it.

The sensations that we go through during childbirth are unlike any other sort of pain. They result in something incredible, and that knowledge helps us to stay focused and strong. Try to hold on to the idea that the pain is temporary and that each new contraction

Sam: "When I found out I was pregnant for the second time I was filled with joy. However, my fears soon hit me. What if I had another premature baby? I decided to practise yoga daily and do a course on hypnobirthing to calm my nerves, and my fears subsided. In the end I gave birth to Yasmin in less than four hours with no pain relief."

brings you closer to meeting your baby. Whether you give birth vaginally or have a c-section, the focus should firmly stay on meeting your new baby for the first time.

This fear often means that women are scared to really learn about birth. They feel they have no option but to turn up at hospital when their contractions are strong enough and be directed by the medical team. But doctors and midwives can be restricted by time pressures and may sometimes suggest what is convenient for them and the hospital. Remember that the medical team won't have the chance to really get to know you, and so unless you have a strong vision of what you want, they may make assumptions. It is important to listen to medical advice, but if you have any preferences about the sort of birth, pain relief and birthing positions that you are hoping for, it is wise to communicate this.

The most important aspect of your birthing story is to believe that you can do it. Always remember that labour is finite, and every second of it is leading to an extraordinary new chapter in your life.

Prepare for all eventualities

Childbirth cannot be meticulously planned. Your baby will take the time they needs to emerge, your cervix will open at its own rate, your contractions will set their own rhythm. Moving with it, adopting positions that encourage the process, using your breath to give you energy and focus, finding natural ways to relieve the contractions, will all help your labour to progress. A birth plan is not a list of instructions to dictate your birth story. You need to be flexible and open to possibilities.

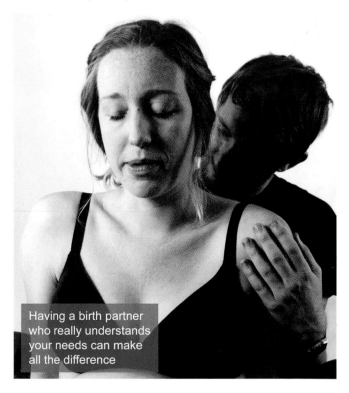

Having a birth partner who really understands your needs can make all the difference

A natural birth may well be your first choice, but if your own health or that of your child's is at risk then a c-section can be a safer way to deliver your baby. Your main purpose should be to do whatever keeps your baby safe and healthy. If your child is not getting enough oxygen, then delivery by ventouse (suction cup) or forceps can be helpful. These assisted delivery options are also used if you feel exhausted and unable to push anymore, the baby's head needs turning, the baby is distressed or the baby is struggling to find their way through the pelvis. Drugs may help speed the labour along, freeing up the staff and the room you are in, but they may make you feel out of control. Alternatively, an epidural may be the best solution for you in your changing circumstances.

It's great to feel at peace with all of the options before you enter the delivery suite.

Find a birth partner who can act as your voice

A birth partner may not be your life partner; they could be a close friend or a family member, or even a doula. However, they need to be someone who listens to you, who is able to stand their ground and who is self-sufficient. They should not be someone you might be worried about during the labour. Talk about what you want from the birthing experience and explain the stages of labour to your birth partner. You may have spent a great deal of time writing your birth plan, but your midwife or birthing team may not have the time to read through your plan in detail. Having

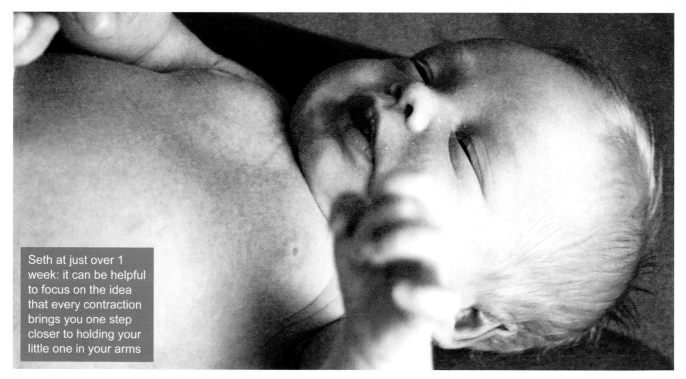

Seth at just over 1 week: it can be helpful to focus on the idea that every contraction brings you one step closer to holding your little one in your arms

a birth partner who can voice your opinion and act as your advocate can be hugely beneficial. Your birth partner can help you to make a rational decision about pain relief and assisted labour. They can listen to the medical team and assess the ongoing situation while you focus on breathing deeply and following your instincts.

The stages of labour

Knowing exactly what your body goes through will help you to make informed decisions as well as preparing you for the birthing process.

Oxytocin plays a key role in childbirth. Contractions are caused by rising levels in oxytocin, which peak just before you give birth. Oxytocin also helps a mother to push out the placenta, and causes the womb to gradually shrink back after birth. Oxytocin plays a key part in the letdown reflex, enabling the breasts to make milk.

The first stage of labour

Medical teams find examination easier when a woman is lying on her back, but this posture closes up the pelvis, which can make it harder for the baby to squeeze through. Ideally, you want to be as upright as possible, keeping your pelvis open to allow gravity to assist you with the birthing process.

The first stage is when your cervix gradually opens. This stage is divided into three distinct parts: early labour, active labour and the transitional stage. The first stage of labour can last 6-20 hours, or 2-10 hours if it isn't a first-time labour.[1] It can be difficult to distinguish between the three stages, particularly if this is your first labour.

Your cervix starts off in a posterior position (pointing towards your back) and during early labour it will move to an anterior position (towards your front). It will also soften and shorten. As your cervix adjusts you may feel a slight backache or mild abdominal aches; you may even have loose bowels. This stage is sometimes referred to as pre-labour. During the first stage your cervix will eventually open until it is fully dilated (10cm/4" in diameter).

During pregnancy a mucus plug forms over the cervix to keep infection out, and before labour this plug comes away. This jelly-like substance (which may be a little blood-stained) is known as a show. For first labours the show usually signifies that labour is coming within hours or days. If you've given birth before, then your show could be a sign that you are already in labour.

■ Early labour

This is the stage in which your cervix goes from being closed to 3-4cm (1⅛-1⅝") dilated. Some women don't realize it has started, though the intensity of contractions will increase. It often feels like a period pain, with mild cramps and/or a dull backache. At this stage it is worth timing your contractions. In early labour they are erratic and often

---

Sam: "During the first stage of labour I'd recommend a bath with some lavender oil. The essential oil will soothe your nervous system and help relax you and your baby, while the warm water will help to release oxytocin ready for your birth."

more than 5 minutes apart, lasting 30-40 seconds. Once they have fallen into a steady pattern, closer together and lasting longer, you are in true labour.

During this early stage you should be able to talk and move around. You might want to phone parents or close friends and make any last-minute arrangements, ensure other children are taken care of and gather your hospital bag together. If you are planning a hospital birth, it is advisable to stay at home. Early labour can stop and start, and going into hospital can actually delay the labour. You are better off trying to relax in a familiar environment. This is a good time to drink plenty of water and eat something nutritious. You may not feel like much, but your body will need the energy later and you may not be able to eat for a while. Complex carbs, protein and minerals are all important. So even a slice or two of wholemeal toast, a glass of milk and some fruit would be helpful.

This is the ideal time for a warm bath or some meditation or mindfulness exercises. Some women find that staying upright helps with the discomfort, so you might like to keep walking.

■ The active phase

This is the phase when your cervix opens to 10cm (4") and it lasts for 2-3½ hours on average. Your contractions will become stronger, longer and more frequent, occurring every 3 to 4 minutes and lasting 40-60 seconds. It is likely that you won't be able to talk through them now. This can seem quite intense as there is little time to rest between contractions. Focus on the idea that each one is helping your baby out into this world.

Keep your body as relaxed as possible during this time. Instead of trying to talk, focus on your breathing. You may find some comfort in rocking gently on a birthing ball. This will not only ease the pain but can also help to keep the pelvis supple and open.

Most women will head to the hospital, if that is where they are having their baby, between the first two phases of labour – as the early phase ends and the active phase begins.[2]

It's best to ring the maternity unit and let them know you will be arriving. The midwife may want to speak to you to get a sense of how progressed your labour is. If you go into hospital too early, it is possible that they will send you home. It is advisable to stay at home for as long as possible as you will feel more relaxed there, which will help the labour to progress. During this stage it is likely that you will find it difficult to move during contractions.

Some women feel anxious about giving birth in the car on the way to the hospital, or if they are having a home birth, they worry that the midwife will not show up on time. Both scenarios are rare. Think of all the babies you know: how many of them were born in a car or before the midwife arrived? With good preparation in the third trimester and a reliable birth partner in place who has familiarized themselves with the stages of labour, all you need to do now is focus on your breathing. The calmer you are, the more oxytocin will flow, and the shorter and simpler your labour is likely to be. Always remember how many billions of women have given birth successfully before you.

■ The transitional phase

This is the stage between your cervix becoming fully dilated and the urge to push, and on average this lasts from 15 minutes to an hour. Contractions tend to be less frequent but last longer and may be more intense. Sometimes a contraction will start before the last one has fully faded. It is common for your waters to break during or before this phase. Some women find this phase almost overwhelming, and it is really important to remind yourself that it signifies the full opening of the cervix. Often there is a break from contractions before the pushing stage.

The transitional phase is often the hardest stage of labour so use pain relief if you need it. Gas and air can take the edge off the intensity, although some women find that experiencing the heaviest contractions without it actually encourages them to push, thereby leading to a shorter labour.

The second stage of labour

This is the stage in which you will push your baby down the birth canal. Keeping your pelvis open is essential, so avoid lying on your back if you can. If you stay upright, gravity will assist you. Squatting positions are really helpful, as is kneeling on all fours. Whichever position you are in, it is helpful to move around. Rotate your hips in a figure of eight, sway and keep active. This will give your baby the space to find a suitable position.

If you want to lie down (because you need to rest or have had an epidural), lie on one side and ask your birth partner to support your upper leg to relieve any pressure on the lower back.

The second stage of labour usually doesn't last more than a couple of hours. Sometimes it only takes minutes. With subsequent babies it can be as little as 5-10 minutes.

When you feel the urge to push you can bear down, listen to your body and work with your contractions. In between contractions be sure to breathe deeply and slowly. It is common to make some noise when you are actively pushing, so embrace the urge to roar or shout and please don't be embarrassed. Follow your primal instincts. (Remember the noises that body builders make when they are lifting huge weights?) Making noise can actually help you to relax, whereas suppressing the natural urge to be vocal can cause tension and slow this stage down. With each push your baby will slowly move a little bit further down your vagina.

Crowning is when your vagina stretches over the baby's head. Your midwife will be looking out for this. You will feel a hot stinging sensation. At this point you need to stop pushing and pant lightly: your midwife will tell you when to do this, so listen for their instructions. This will allow your baby to be born as gently as possible, making it less traumatic for them, and less likely that you will tear. Sometimes the head is born in one contraction and the body in the other. It may happen in one smooth movement. The moment when your baby emerges from your body has to be one of the most awe-inspiring moments of anyone's life. You may want to look; you may want to shut your eyes and focus on summoning up every drop of energy for that last big push. When the baby has slipped into the world, all the intensity will stop as if by magic, and you will probably be speechless. As will your birth partner. If the second stage of labour was very quick, you may be shaking all over with adrenalin (which your body produces to give you the energy to push). But hold on – there's still more ...

The third stage of labour

This is when you deliver the placenta and membranes. Once the baby is born you may only have a few moments of rest before your body starts to contract again in order to expel these.

You can have an injection that will mean you don't need to push – this will create contractions. Some women opt for this as they may feel completely wiped out (especially if they had an unusually short or long labour) and simply want to get the third stage over with quickly, so that they can focus on their baby. The injection can mean less risk of postnatal anaemia and less bleeding as the placenta is delivered, but can also cause nausea, vomiting and heavier blood loss for several hours.)

Skin-to-skin contact with your newborn and breastfeeding can encourage the third stage. Usually an assisted third

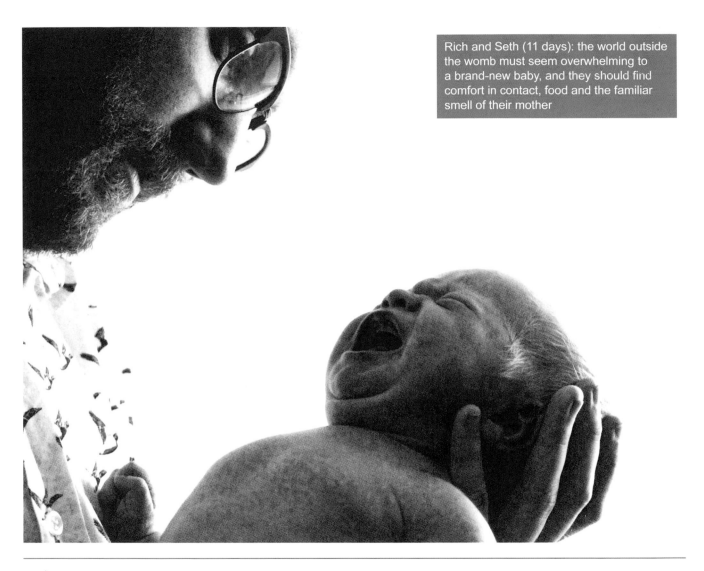

Rich and Seth (11 days): the world outside the womb must seem overwhelming to a brand-new baby, and they should find comfort in contact, food and the familiar smell of their mother

Holly: "I found giving birth to be the most exhilarating experience of my life. Tapping into my instincts, I kept on moving around and used a lot of deep squats. Jasmine was eventually born when I was on all fours, and rocking my pelvis meant she easily found the space to move through."

stage and a natural one (sometimes referred to as a physiological third stage) last the same amount of time, about 5 to 30 minutes.

If you've had a managed third stage, there's more of a chance that you'll need to return to hospital later because of bleeding. This may be due to fragments of placenta or membrane that have been left behind when your midwife eased out the placenta.[3]

Ideally, if there have been no complications, you will keep the umbilical cord attached for a few minutes. This will keep the blood flowing to your baby immediately after the birth.

Active birth positions

Remember, active birth positions rely on gravity to help the baby on the way. Try practising them through pregnancy as they are a lovely way of connecting with your partner, gently strengthening your body and encouraging your muscle memory to learn poses.

These positions should be loose, allowing your muscles to be free of tension and your body to move. Your pelvis should not be constricted in any way. Practise deep breathing while you try out these positions, encouraging the connection between breathing and birthing to become instinctive.

Standing supported squat

Squatting can open up the pelvis by as much as 2cm (about 1"), so is a great position for the second stage of labour. Many women find that contractions in this position are less painful and can increase the urge to push.

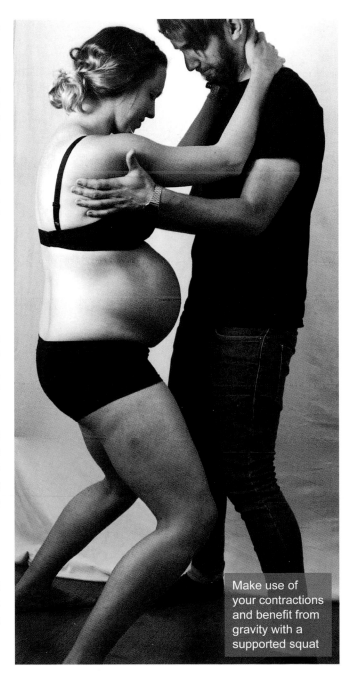

Make use of your contractions and benefit from gravity with a supported squat

The standing supported squat can be done facing away from your partner or facing them. Maintaining eye contact and breathing together can be a nice way to stay connected and for them to help you with your breathing without telling you to breathe! You might like to loop your arm around your partner's neck or hold on to their arms. Alternatively, you could lean against the wall with a gentle bend in your legs.

Maintaining this position can be tiring for both the mum-to-be and her birth partner, so you could break it up with other postures.

Other ways of squatting

You might like to lean against a birthing ball, which allows for a lovely deep squat and gives you plenty of support. It also means that your birth partner is free to massage your back. Squatting between your partner's legs can help you to get into a deep squat. If they sit on the edge of the bed or a chair, you can use your elbows to lean on their legs. It can be helpful to use the fabric of their trousers to pull against as you bear down during contractions, so remind your partner to pack jeans in their hospital bag if you think you might try this position during labour.

Sitting

Straddling a chair means that you can grip the back of the chair during contractions, as well as leaning into it for support. It allows you to rest but still make use of gravity. This can be a useful position if you respond well to massage during labour, as it allows your birth partner access to your whole back. It can also be used with continuous electronic foetal monitoring.

Lying on your side

If it feels like labour is progressing too fast and you just want to take a rest, lying on your side with a pillow or support between your legs is a nice way to have a breather – gravity will slow things down, plus the coccyx (tailbone) isn't closed, which it is if you lie on your back. Your coccyx needs to be able to move freely so that the baby's head has more room to pass through your pelvis.

Lying on your back has other disadvantages. It closes the pelvic outlet by around 20-30 per cent compared to upright positions such as squatting, it makes your birth canal curve upwards, and it can constrict blood vessels. It can also make you feel less in control of your labour.

Walking and standing

Walking, standing and sitting upright (even kneeling) can help you to feel actively involved and speed up labour. But if you have high blood pressure, an upright posture is not advised. When people have high blood pressure their hearts need to work harder. Sitting and standing causes our blood pressure to rise so that the arteries in our hearts and brains continue to receive blood, nutrients and oxygen. In labour our hearts work harder too as adrenalin pumps blood into our muscles. If your blood pressure is already high, it is sensible to try to keep it as stable as possible during labour. These active postures cannot be used with continuous electronic foetal monitoring either. In both scenarios it is better to lie on your side.

On all fours

Whether you opt for a supported kneel (against the bed, with a pile of cushions or a birthing ball) or simply use your hands or forearms to support you, kneeling postures can be restful yet also allow freedom of movement. Many women find a lot of comfort during contractions by rocking backwards and forwards or by making a figure of eight with their hips. Remember that if you keep your hips moving, the baby can find it easier to move through the birth canal. This posture also allows your birth partner access to your back for massage.

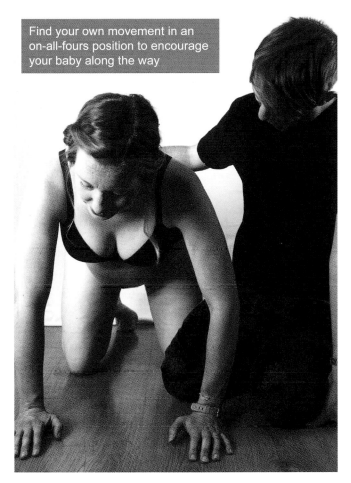

Find your own movement in an on-all-fours position to encourage your baby along the way

Breathing

Remembering to breathe deeply is so important in labour. It will help to keep you calm and collected, and better able to listen to your gut instinct. It will help give you a vital sense of control. It can aid in pain management. It gives you energy, which is so important during childbirth. Breathing properly also helps to supply your baby with plenty of essential oxygen. Counting your breath can help you to time contractions from the start of labour.

Pain makes us naturally tense, our breathing can become shallow and our muscles tight. If our fight-or-flight response is triggered due to fear, this can slow labour down. At the first sign of labour try to loosen your shoulders, keep your spine lengthened and raise your head up. You may feel comfortable walking around, you may prefer to sit. However you position yourself, establishing a deep breathing routine is essential from the outset.

Exhale fully through your mouth, using a long, controlled, measured breath. Count the seconds this takes and then match the seconds as you inhale, keeping that rhythm going for the entire first stage if you can. Every time you breathe out, let your muscles soften: this will help your cervix and vagina to relax too. Once you have established a firm counted breath you may like to add some words, especially if the pain is becoming more intense. It could be a short mantra such as 'I can do this' or 'This too shall pass' (using two words for the inhale and two for the exhale) or you could use one word such as 'relax', breathing in for 're' and out for 'lax'. If you like the sound of a mantra, it might be worth choosing one before you go into labour. Having these little psychological devices to support you can be really empowering!

If you are finding that your breathing is becoming shallow, focus on the out breath (the inhalation will follow naturally). It is worth going through some breathing techniques with your birth partner during the pregnancy as they can help keep you on track. Being told what to do can take away the feeling of empowerment; so rather than telling you to breathe they could gently place their hands on your shoulders, look you in the eye and breathe with you. Perhaps even saying your mantra or counting the breaths for you would work well.

Sometimes using sound can be helpful. Breathe in through your nose as fully as possible and out through your mouth, making a noise as you do so. It may be an 'ooohh' sound or an 'aaahhh'. Sometimes sound can help us to release the pain and deal with it more effectively. This is a useful technique once labour has become established and is progressing well.

You may find that the breathing gives you a dry mouth, so it is a good idea for your birth partner to offer you water regularly. Sometimes sipping water through a straw is helpful so pack some straws and bottles of water in your hospital bag. Again, you may not want to be asked if you would like some water every few minutes so it may be easier for them to simply offer it to you without words or have it on hand so you can point to it if you want it. Being well hydrated will help with breastfeeding, so try to drink as much water as possible during the labour.

Mindfulness

Entering a state of mindfulness can give you the power you need to believe in yourself. You might like to use a pair of words that can keep you positive and focused. You could inhale 'strength' and exhale 'fear' or 'pain'. Coordinating with your breath means it will become instinctual and automatic. Intense contractions may make visualizations such as imagining your vagina opening like a lotus flower impossible to carry out. Instead, keep it simple.

Preparing for an active birth

In the majority of cases, midwives will encourage women to have an active birth. In the Western world, women used to lie on their backs to allow the medical team good access. Nowadays midwives support labours involving upright positions and free movement, and for women in labour to follow their instincts. However, in TV and film dramas there is often a widespread portrayal of women in labour lying on their backs.

The most important preparation for labour is mental. If you are calm, relaxed and confident, then your birth should be quicker and easier. Understanding each of the stages of labour is the first step. It also helps to be armed with your breathing exercises and a number of different techniques – massage, a mantra, a selection of positions, for example – to help you through. Keep an open mind and listen to the signals that your body is giving you.

Writing a birth plan

Your birthing team may never get the opportunity to see your birth plan, or they may skim it. What matters most is that you and your birth partner have written it together and know it inside out. Ideally, your plan should cover every eventuality and will serve as a useful reminder of your wishes. Write it in bullet points that can be quickly

Sam: "I practised mindfulness throughout my second and third labours. Envisioning my baby slowly coming out of me and into the world kept me focused. I felt in control of my body. Overall my labours were an amazing experience."

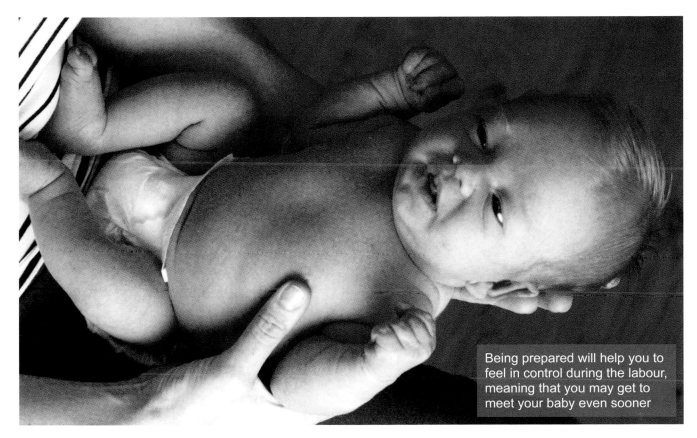

Being prepared will help you to feel in control during the labour, meaning that you may get to meet your baby even sooner

digested and understood. For example, you might ideally want a water birth, but that may depend on the birthing pool's availability or how far your labour has progressed when you are assessed by a midwife. So what's the next best scenario from your point of view?

Some women prefer not to factor in pain relief as it can prolong labour. In that case, you might specify the following under the heading 'pain relief': 'Manage pain through movement, birthing ball, deep breathing and aromatherapy massage. No analgesics [painkilling drugs] if possible. If pain relief needed, gas and air only. Move on to pethidine if essential.'

The topic of pain relief is a sensitive one. During childbirth many women seek to block out the pain signals that their body is giving them with painkilling drugs. These drugs can reach the baby, making breastfeeding harder to establish,[4] and can make some women feel they no longer have control. Many women who have spent a whole nine months avoiding chemicals are reluctant to use drugs in labour. However, if the labour is overly long and exhausting or if the pain becomes too difficult to manage, then painkilling drugs might turn the experience around for you. Giving yourself permission on your birth plan to be flexible if the situation demands, and working out what feels right for you, will help you to maintain an all-important sense of control.

Painkilling-drug options

As with all aspects of the birthing process, it is worth knowing about the different types of pain-relieving drugs before you go into the delivery suite.

Entonox (gas and air)

This is a mixture of 50 per cent oxygen and 50 per cent nitrous oxide gas. It won't kill the pain but can make it feel more manageable. Gas and air is the most popular method of pain relief used in labour. It should be readily available in maternity units and from a registered midwife during a home birth. As a new contraction starts, you take in gas and air through an antibacterial filter using a mouthpiece or mask which you hold yourself. The mouthpiece has a two-way valve that releases the gas and air and takes away the carbon dioxide that you breathe out. You continue to breathe deeply and evenly, in and out, for around 15-20 seconds until you start to feel a little light-headed, then you take the mouthpiece away from your face. Within a few seconds you'll feel normal again.[5]

Entonox crosses the placental barrier and high doses of it can affect your body's vitamin B12 levels as well as cell development.[6] A study in the *British Medical Journal* in 1990 found that the children of women who had used entonox for longer and more often during their labours than during their labours of their siblings were more likely to develop an amphetamine addiction in later life.[7]

Using gas and air means that you can control it yourself, it is quite easy to use and you can stop taking it whenever you want. The mixture makes some women feel queasy, and it can also give you a dry mouth, dizziness and cause confusion. On the other hand, entonox can offset anxiety, helps you to focus on your breathing and may take the edge off the intensity of your contractions and hence avoid the need for an epidural.

Pethidine

Pethidine is given as a single intramuscular injection (usually into the buttock or thigh). About 25 per cent of women use an opioid such as pethidine in labour in the UK.[8]

It takes between twenty minutes and four hours to take effect. Your midwife will advise you when to have the injection as if it is given too close to the end of labour, you may find it hard to push. It can also affect the baby's breathing if it is administered too late in the labour. Some women start off with a half dose. Pethidine can cause nausea and confusion, and can also make some babies struggle with their first feed. Pethidine will allow you to move around, which is not always possible with an epidural.

Epidural or spinal

Epidurals or spinals, regional anaesthetics that usually provide complete pain relief, are used by about a third of women in labour in the UK,[9] and in a limited study over 27 states, 61 per cent of women in the USA.[10] In a recent report, the epidural rate in Canada varied between provinces from 30 to 69 per cent.[11] It is estimated that epidurals are administered in approximately 25 per cent of all labours in New Zealand.[12] A decade ago, Australia's caesarean rate was only 19 per cent; now it's 32 per cent.[13]

These drugs are administered by an anaesthetist (so are not an option for home births) and block the pain impulses from the birth canal to the brain (by numbing the nerves).

In some hospitals they can offer mobile epidurals that allow you some movement. These rely on remote monitoring of the baby's heart rate, but many hospitals are unable to give them because they don't have the specialist staff to ensure that it is safe for you to move about. You may find that you only have a very limited amount of movement. Some women can manage to move from the bed to a chair, and a few can walk with help.[14]

Many women assume that by opting for an epidural they will have all the pain relief that they will need, but according to the UK-based Obstetrics Anaesthetists' Association, one in eight women who have an epidural during labour need to use other forms of pain relief.[15]

The main difference between a spinal and an epidural is that a full spinal works faster, but it only lasts about two hours and cannot be topped up.[16] The downside to epidurals and spinals, aside from the risk of a severe headache if fluid from the spine leaks, is that they may stop the oxytocin levels building during labour.[17] Women who have an epidural may find that the pushing stage of labour lasts longer and there is a greater chance of needing help via forceps or a ventouse.[18]

Epidurals are known to have a negative impact on breastfeeding for the first 24 hours of a baby's life (even though they don't inhibit the percentage of breastfeeding attempts in the first hour)[19] and like any medication used during labour will enter the baby's bloodstream through the umbilical cord.[20] This painkilling option can also take away the feeling of being in control of the labour process away from the mother. According to the UK *Observer* newspaper, Professor Denis Walsh (one of Britain's most influential midwives) claimed that "pain-relieving drugs, including epidural injections, carry serious medical risks, diminish childbirth as a rite of passage and undermine the mother's bond with her child".[21]

What to consider on your birth plan

- Your birth partner
- Monitoring (continuous electronic monitoring can hinder freedom of movement so in some cases it is essential)
- Interventions (are you happy to be given a drug to speed up the labour if it slows down?)
- Assisted delivery (what are your thoughts on forceps and ventouse and will you rely on the midwife's opinion on the day?)
- Birthing positions (list several options)
- Managed or physiological third stage (a managed third stage of labour means having an injection to trigger contractions so you don't have to push the placenta out yourself)
- Breastfeeding: if for any reason you don't wish to breastfeed at birth, include this in your plan. Globally, 44 per cent of babies breastfeed within an hour of being born, but only 39 per cent of babies benefit from exclusive breastfeeding between birth and 5 months.[22] Unicef say that virtually every mother can breastfeed, if given appropriate support, advice and encouragement, as well as practical assistance to resolve any problems[23]
- Delayed cord clamping? Delaying the cutting of the umbilical cord until after

{cont.}

pulsations have stopped or the placenta has been delivered is recommended by the World Health Organization as it can lower the risk of anaemia[24] and increase blood volume, and because the placental blood is so rich in stem cells.[25] There are more stem cells in your baby's foetal blood than at any other time in their life, and they play a vital part in your baby's development including the cardiovascular, respiratory, immune and central nervous systems.[26] As iron deficiency anaemia affects both the physical and the cognitive development of children,[27] delayed cord clamping is highly recommended. Some midwives will cut the cord early out of habit, so be sure to speak out or ask your birth partner to. Your birth partner may even wish to cut the cord themselves

- Some women would rather their baby was cleaned up before being handed to them; others are keen for instant skin-to-skin contact

- State whatever feels right for you and include it in the plan. Your birthing team will have seen all sorts of labours. If you have any special needs, including dietary needs or health issues, it is important to include them especially if you are planning on giving birth in hospital.

Birthing options
Elective caesarean

In some cases you will be advised to have a planned caesarean because of previous complications during birth or an underlying medical issue. For many women, there may be an emotional or psychological motive. Others opt for one because their previous birthing experience was too distressing.

In 2015, the World Health Organization issued new guidelines for elective or planned caesareans. From 1985 on, the international healthcare community has considered the ideal rate for caesarean sections to be between 10 and 15 per cent. But since then, caesarean sections have become increasingly common in both developed and developing countries. When medically necessary, a caesarean section can effectively prevent maternal and newborn mortality.[28] However, there is no evidence that shows the benefits of caesarean delivery for women or infants who did not medically require the procedure. Although caesarean section has become a very safe procedure in many parts of the world, it is not without risk.[29]

A c-section can mean a substantially delayed recovery period, and for some women, planning to have a natural birth only to find that a caesarean is necessary, it can be traumatic. Other women are criticized when they opt for an elective caesarean. Although many women go on to have vaginal births after a caesarean, there are others who

Holly: "As my labour progressed so quickly my birth plan stayed in my hospital bag, but having written it meant that my birth partner knew exactly what I wanted. Writing the plan made me aware of my options and all possible outcomes, which helped me to feel in control."

are faced with the same physiological issues they had the first time round. Choosing one after a traumatic first birth can be an important way of regaining control and feeling positive about your birthing experience.

You know your body and you know what you will feel comfortable with. No one should feel any pressure to put their child or their own health at risk.

Reasons for a home birth

For many couples, a home birth seems like a wise choice. If you have enjoyed a healthy pregnancy and have no health complications, then giving birth at home may make you feel more relaxed. In some cases, your doctor or midwife may advise you to give birth in a hospital. If you have any health concerns or are over 35, then there is a possibility that your doctor may advise against home birth.

One of the greatest advantages of giving birth at home is that your familiar surroundings should trigger the all-important oxytocin that really helps when you are giving birth. Oxytocin levels will build during the labour (and are instrumental in achieving powerful contractions). Oxytocin can calm you down and when it peaks at delivery it can also give you an intense feeling of euphoria. High levels of oxytocin after the birth will help you to bond with your baby, as well as encouraging the letdown reflex that is essential for breastfeeding.

Being surrounded by your own belongings and knowing that everything that you could possibly need is on hand has real advantages. Being able to play your own music, use your own birthing pool or having easy access to ice can also make a big difference. Most women get quite hot during the active stage of labour; adding several flannels to a bowl of water and ice means you will always have a cool, refreshing cloth to hand. Sitting on ice packs can also bring relief after a vaginal delivery. You can control the temperature, create an atmosphere that feels appropriate

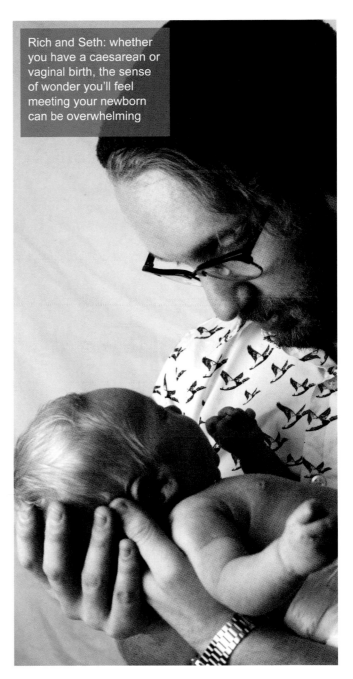

Rich and Seth: whether you have a caesarean or vaginal birth, the sense of wonder you'll feel meeting your newborn can be overwhelming

and follow your instincts. Many women like the idea of not having to factor in the physical journey to the hospital or the possibility that they might be sent home, which can help to reduce any anxieties they have around the labour.

If you decide on a home birth, then your midwife will talk through the options with you. Your midwife may not be on duty when you go into labour, so they will leave everything they need for the birth at your house in preparation.

Many women prefer a home birth in principle but may be put off by the fact that painkilling drugs, if suddenly required, won't be available to fall back on, or by the prospect of a bloody mess. In fact, part of the midwife's role is to tidy up the mess. They will bring disposable pads and will dispose of the afterbirth too. You might like to place protective sheeting (even a shower curtain or waterproof tablecloth) and some old sheets on your bed. Many women use a waterproof mattress cover towards the end of pregnancy in case their waters break during the night.

Practicalities of a home birth

The number of midwives who attend to you during a home birth varies depending on where you live. In your area you may be allocated two midwives. Your midwife will give you full details of how to contact them when you go into labour. They will also advise you if they feel that you should go to the hospital at any stage during the labour.

Midwives in the UK are under a professional duty of care to attend your birth if you choose to have a home birth, and are legally obliged to do all that they can to attend your birth. If they are unable to attend, then they are obliged to find a replacement midwife, and in most areas there is a second midwife on call in place. In America, the laws vary from state to state and in some areas home-birthing is restricted. Certified professional midwives are only allowed to practise in 28 states, and in some states a direct-entry midwife (an independent practitioner) is not allowed to attend a home birth unless a medical doctor is present. The Midwives Alliance of North America referred to this as 'archaic'.[30] In some Canadian provinces, where midwifery is legislated and legal, midwives can attend your labour and birth in your own home.[31] In New Zealand a pregnant women can choose between giving birth at home, in hospital or in a birthing centre (which is a small maternity unit staffed by midwives). She is even allowed to choose her lead maternity carer (LMC), who will provide a complete and consistent maternity service from pregnancy until after the baby is 4-6 weeks old.[32] The option to give birth at home is uncertain for Australian women, due to current issues around private indemnity insurance for privately practising midwives.[33]

It is worth having a good chat with your midwife about all the options well before you are due to give birth. If a home birth is not possible, then there are plenty of other ways to feel in control and relaxed during your labour. Sorting out all of the practical aspects of the birth, such as insurance, with plenty of time to spare means that you will feel calmer as your due date approaches.

Holly: "I would have loved to have had a home birth but my partner encouraged me to opt for the local hospital. In the end, Jasmine's birth was such a positive experience that it didn't really matter where it happened, but in future, I'd prefer to give birth at home."

Holly: "I was desperate for a water birth – I can easily spend hours in the bath and it felt like a really soothing option. However, a birthing pool takes a while to fill and my labour developed very quickly. So if you fancy a water birth, whether at home or in hospital, I'd ask your birthing partner or team to fill your pool as soon as possible."

Water birth

Warm water is not only a gentle means of pain relief, but it also helps you feel relaxed and calm by encouraging the release of oxytocin. It allows you your own personal space. Your birth partner could come in the pool too if you invite them to.

For a baby who is used to living in a watery environment, being born into water can be a more natural transition. Using a birthing pool during the second stage of labour can help ease contractions. You may choose to give birth in the pool, you may prefer dry land.

Many women like the idea of being submerged in the comfort and privacy of water yet worry that the water will become bloody. As it is the placenta that is the most bloody, you could choose to deliver the placenta on the bed. However you look at it there will be blood during labour.

Gentle pain-relief during labour

Massage

Massage is a wonderful way for your birth partner to feel connected to you without words. Even the most verbose of us may fall silent during labour, with the exception of some gutteral roars!

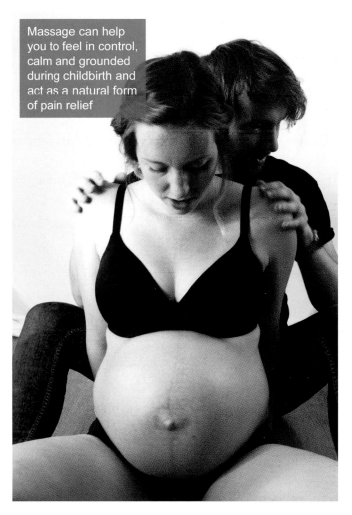

Massage can help you to feel in control, calm and grounded during childbirth and act as a natural form of pain relief

It can be helpful if your partner focuses on your lower back, using the heel of their hand to draw firm circles on the pelvis. Large, slow, soothing strokes may be more effective. They could even coordinate the strokes with your breathing to encourage slow, deep breaths, moving their hands from coccyx to neck with each inhalation, and stroking down the back as you breathe out.

Smell the roses, blow out the candles

Breathe in deeply through your nose (imagine you are smelling something beautiful such as a rose garden) for four counts, then breathe out slowly through a small opening in your mouth (as if blowing out a candle) for eight counts.

This is a lovely breathing exercise that can be used in pregnancy too, increasing oxygen flow to your baby and making you feel more relaxed. The idea is to breathe out for double the time that you breathe in. If you are heavily pregnant, shorten the time to six counts (and breathe in for three). The idea is not to count for as long as possible, just to find a breathing pattern that works for you. It is a good idea to practise this breathing technique several times a day, especially when stressed. Even if you are not pregnant, the advantages of using breath control are many.

Hypnobirthing

Hypnobirthing involves using self-hypnosis, breathing techniques and relaxation strategies to encourage women to feel more in control and confident during childbirth.

The thinking behind hypnobirthing is that by following her natural instincts, a woman will be more at ease. If you are able to reach a deep level of relaxation, then your muscles will be more pliant and childbirth will be much easier. When you are tense and stressed, the muscles of your body may become rigid. This includes the muscles in your vagina, meaning that your body is resisting its natural urge to open up. Tension will also mean that you tire more easily and have less energy. Deep breathing is a great way to get energy into the body, as well as oxygen into the muscles to give them greater power. When we are in pain, most of us take shallow breaths. By learning to breathe deeply throughout pregnancy you will find it easier to take deep nurturing breaths throughout labour.

Massage oil blend for labour

Avoid sweet almond carrier oil in case your newborn-to-be has a nut allergy. Rose and jasmine essential oil should only be handled once labour has started and not during pregnancy.

100ml (3½fl oz) carrier oil
  (wheatgerm, jojoba or grapeseed)
5 drops of lavender essential oil
5 drops of rose essential oil
5 drops of jasmine essential oil

Mix them together and store out of direct sunlight. Shake the bottle gently before use to disperse the essential oils.

Some women find that they don't want to be touched during labour, in which case you can add a drop of lavender, rose and jasmine to a handkerchief and inhale directly. You can also add two drops of each oil to an oil burner with a teaspoon of water if you are giving birth at home or during the early stages of labour. You can buy electronic oil diffusers although a battery-operated one may be easier in hospital.

TENS machine

TENS (transcutaneous electrical nerve stimulation) machines work by interrupting and reducing pain signals as they travel to the brain. You attach the sticky pads (or electrodes) directly to your skin and adjust the intensity of the electrical flow. They can be very effective as a means of mild pain management, particularly in early labour, and can stimulate the production of endorphins. As TENS machines are battery operated and the device is small and easy to operate, you can also clip a TENS machine on to your belt or put it in the pocket of a dressing gown. However, if you move around a lot or want to step in and out of a bath, it may only be useful for a short while.

Birthing realities

Some elements of the birthing experience are glossed over. Here are some of the aspects that we feel you might like to be prepared for:

Contractions

Squeezing your baby out through your vagina is what most women worry about, but the muscles in the area are built to expand and allow the baby through. Staying upright to let gravity give you a helping hand is usually your best option. Contractions can spread through the lower back, abdomen, hips and thighs and can be very intense and exhausting. This is why it is so useful to use breathing exercises to co ordinate with your contractions and to remind yourself that you should be grateful for each breath, as it is helping your baby make their way into the world.

Blood

The media portrayal of labour is as clean albeit painful. The blood will look dramatic, especially if soaking into white hospital sheets. This is why it is important to keep an eye on your iron levels after the birth. Blood loss during birth is rarely more than 500ml (17-18fl oz), but it can seem like a lot at the time.

Poo

Your baby's head will push against your bowels, and combined with you pushing down this can cause many women to poo during labour. This is perfectly natural and your birthing team will have seen it all before. They will simply remove it to keep the area clean. If this happens, you will likely be too consumed by the birth to feel embarrassed. If you feel the urge to go, don't resist it or this may hinder the birthing progress.

Waters breaking

Many women assume that their waters will break in a sudden and dramatic burst that will signify the start of labour. In films this can be a visual way to portray childbirth. In reality the waters usually break around the transitional stage and it is often more of a steady trickle than a sudden burst. If your waters haven't broken and you are ready to push, your midwife may use a small plastic hook to rupture the amniotic membrane. This is a pain-free procedure.

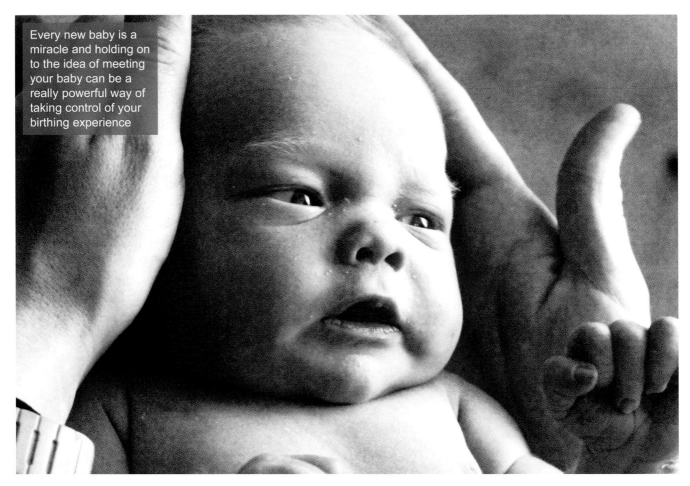

Every new baby is a miracle and holding on to the idea of meeting your baby can be a really powerful way of taking control of your birthing experience

Final thoughts

You are far more brilliant than you realize. Whether this is your first baby or your fifth; whether you give birth vaginally or via c-section; whether you opt for a home birth or a hospital stay; hire a doula or have your mum there to hold your hand; each birth story is unique and beautiful, just like your child will be, and just like your bond with that child will be. So listen to what other parents have to say and digest the advice you get from health professionals. Above all, remember that you have lived in your body for many years and you know yourself and what will work for you.

As soon as you announce you are pregnant people will start giving you advice, and this will continue through each stage of your child's development. So make your own well-informed decisions and go with what feels right for you and your child.

Welcome to parenthood, where the happiest parents leave their preconceptions at the door!

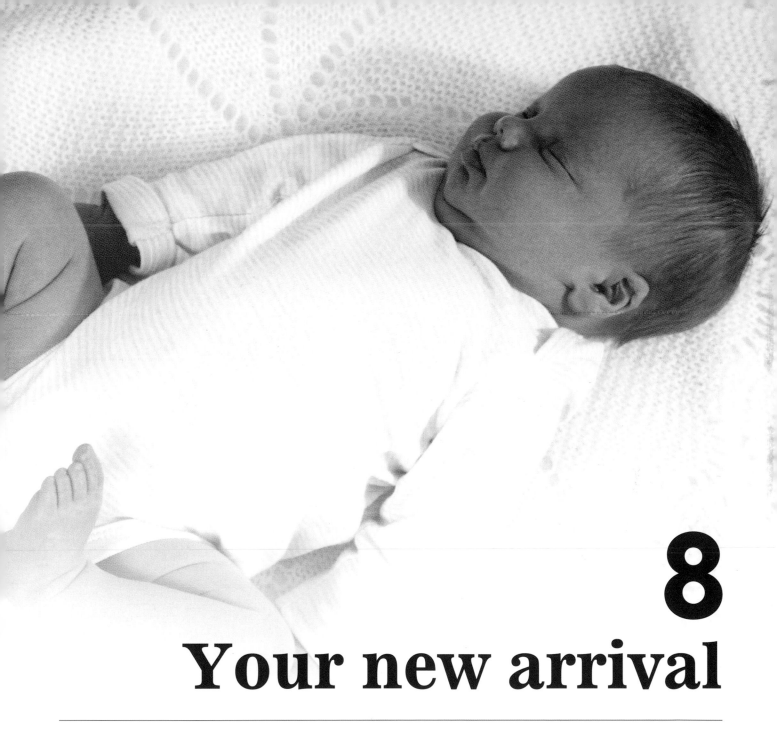

8

Your new arrival

8
Your new arrival

After all the months of waiting and dreaming it is incredibly exciting when your baby is finally born, but it also takes time and effort for parents to get to know their newborn and for the newborn to adjust to their new world. For most parents getting to know their child is commonly known as bonding. In other words, you fall head over heels in love with your baby.

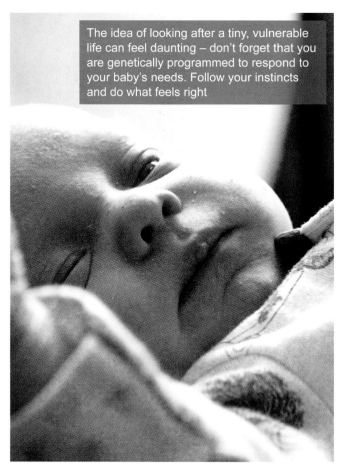

The idea of looking after a tiny, vulnerable life can feel daunting – don't forget that you are genetically programmed to respond to your baby's needs. Follow your instincts and do what feels right

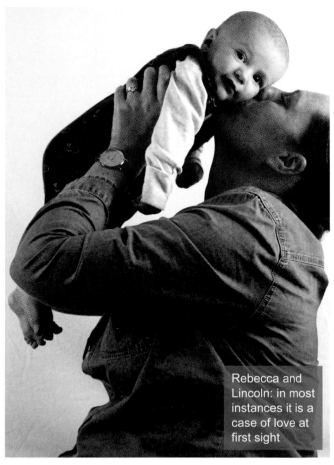

Rebecca and Lincoln: in most instances it is a case of love at first sight

Bonding is triggered by the hormone dopamine that is rushing through your body after you give birth, making you want to protect that tiny child with every fibre of your being. Our parental instinct makes us want to give them everything they need and love them unconditionally forever. This hormone is also what helps your baby to connect emotionally to you.[1] However, a few days after giving birth there is a sudden drop in hormones such as oestrogen and progesterone, which can cause a depression-inducing chemical imbalance in your brain. During pregnancy, levels of progesterone in a woman's body are at their highest, and progesterone has a calming effect.[2] When levels of this hormone drop, it can cause feelings of anxiety and depression. While it is normal to suffer moodswings known as 'the baby blues' during the first few weeks after birth, it could be a sign of postnatal depression if these symptoms don't clear up. If you are feeling low, it's a good idea to speak with your midwife.

The bonding process usually starts during pregnancy so that by the time the birth does come around, you almost can't wait to see your child. This excitement also helps to (literally) push labour on, making it quicker.

For some, bonding takes time, and this can cause worry and stress. It can be a daunting task, realizing that this tiny infant will rely solely on you for everything, and otherwise is totally helpless – it can scare the bonding away for a while as you try to come to terms with what has happened, and how different your life will be from this point on.

Sometimes it takes a few months to adjust to this new way of life, and to this new person who is now taking over so much of what went before. Don't worry. Perhaps the

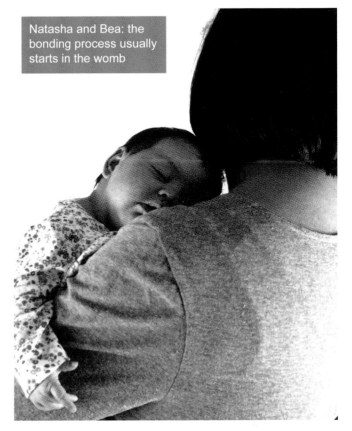

Natasha and Bea: the bonding process usually starts in the womb

labour was a long one, and you are physically exhausted, so much so that your own body needs to rest before you are able to feel anything much for anyone. Maybe it was a long hard pregnancy, or maybe you are worried that you won't be able to care for the little one. Your partner could be having trouble adjusting to their new commitment and the fact that they no longer come first. All of this can affect those initial moments of bonding, and happens to many people every day – you are not alone.

Holly: "For many women the bond grows over time. It's important to give yourself the space to process your emotions."

Twins can make bonding that much harder, especially if one requires additional support following birth. This can bring about feelings of guilt that you are bonding with one and not the other. The same goes for any child who needs to be cared for in a neonatal unit after birth. Seeing your child in person or even in a photo can help. Expressing milk is another way to bond.

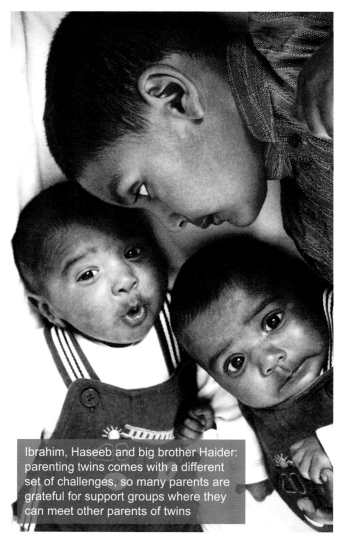

Ibrahim, Haseeb and big brother Haider: parenting twins comes with a different set of challenges, so many parents are grateful for support groups where they can meet other parents of twins

Whether bonding comes easily to you or not, taking a 'babymoon' will give you the time you need with your newborn to help the bonding process. A babymoon is a nesting period of around six weeks, to allow a new mum to recover from the birth properly, during which you are with your baby all the time. It may be difficult to sustain time with just your baby, particularly if you have other children, but take every opportunity you can to rest together in a quiet space. For example, if your employer invites you to your workplace to show off your newborn, feel free to politely refuse without a shred of guilt. Using all the techniques we cover in this chapter, including baby massage, your bonding experience should be something to savour.

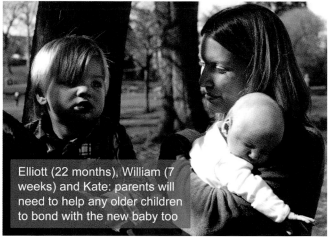

Elliott (22 months), William (7 weeks) and Kate: parents will need to help any older children to bond with the new baby too

How can I help the bonding process?

Skin-to-skin contact is a wonderful way to begin and can start as soon as your baby is born when they are placed on your chest. To your child, your smell is totally unique, and they will sense who you are and what you represent. Babies learn their mother's smell early in life, wiring the scent into their brains.[3]

Breastfeeding is another way to bond, and your midwife will usually encourage you to begin this soon after the birth. Straight after labour your breasts are full of colostrum, which is high in protein, fat-soluble vitamins and antibodies that protect your baby and support their immune system.

Your transitional milk replaces colostrum two to four days after childbirth. If you are wondering when it will appear, try some skin-to-skin contact with your baby, perhaps by placing them on your uncovered breasts, to encourage the milk to flow. A few weeks after that your mature milk comes in. This will be thinner and contain more water than transitional milk. There are two types of mature milk: foremilk occurs at the beginning of the feeding and contains more water, and hindmilk comes at the end of a feed when the breast is nearly empty and contains higher levels of fat.[4]

Sometimes it is not possible to hold your baby immediately after they are is born because of the birth itself (perhaps it was a caesarean) or because the baby needs extra care (perhaps they were premature). This can cause upset for some mothers, but there is no need to worry, as there is no window of time for bonding. You may begin to bond through pregnancy, or as soon as you can hold your baby, even if that is minutes, hours, days or even weeks after the birth itself.

Keeping your baby physically close to you will encourage bonding. Babies need constant reassurance in this scary new world of theirs, and this is the perfect way to do it. It also gives you a chance to learn about your baby, to understand the non-verbal cues they are giving, so that in the future you may be able to attend to their needs before they even begin to cry.

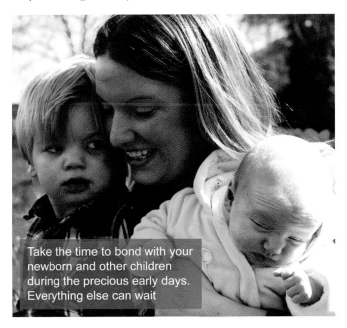

Take the time to bond with your newborn and other children during the precious early days. Everything else can wait

Skin-to-skin contact

Skin-to-skin contact between parents and their newborn babies can provide a wealth of health and emotional benefits. Research has shown that contact after birth and in the days, weeks and months that follow can have a huge impact on your baby's heart rate and sense of well-being, and in strengthening the bond between baby and parent.[5]

Sam: "Ella's birth was traumatic, so it took me a few weeks to get over the shock and really start to relax and bond with her. I feel it depends on the nature of the pregnancy, birth and support you have as to how your bonding experience begins."

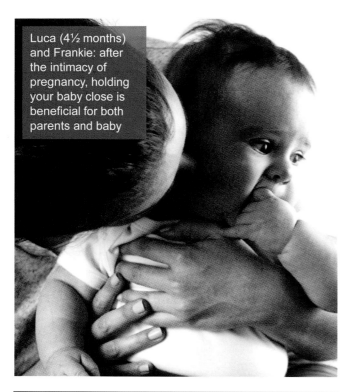

Luca (4½ months) and Frankie: after the intimacy of pregnancy, holding your baby close is beneficial for both parents and baby

For premature babies, the effects can be astounding. Skin-to-skin contact is sometimes referred to as kangaroo care and is often carried out for prolonged periods in the special-care units at hospital. Premature babies are able to regulate their temperatures just as well as they would inside an incubator.

So as your baby's skin is such a vital tool for bonding with you, it's really important to look after it.

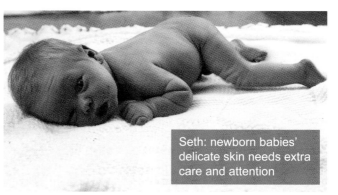

Seth: newborn babies' delicate skin needs extra care and attention

Benefits of skin-to-skin

- Helps to stabilize your baby's temperature, heart rate and breathing
- Allows a baby to colonize their mother's bacteria (immediately after birth), essential for the prevention of allergies developing
- Forms a bond between baby and parent
- Reduces stress levels of both baby and parent
- facilitates breastfeeding.

Caring for newborn skin

Your newborn baby's skin is very different from your own, and it deserves a little extra attention to keep it soft and smooth. Everything that you put on to your baby's skin is absorbed much more quickly, so choose products carefully.

Look for natural and organic products that have been endorsed by the Soil Association (these are certified natural products with the highest-quality ingredients), and look for organic cotton too. No chemicals are used on organic clothing, which helps to reduce the risk of irritation.

Always use non-bio washing products to wash your baby's clothes, or opt for organic laundry detergents.

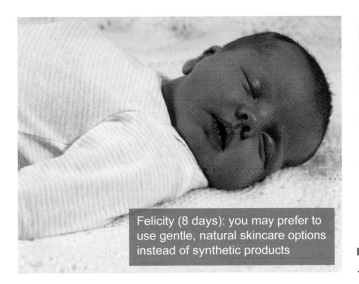

Felicity (8 days): you may prefer to use gentle, natural skincare options instead of synthetic products

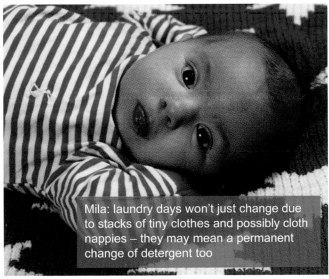

Mila: laundry days won't just change due to stacks of tiny clothes and possibly cloth nappies – they may mean a permanent change of detergent too

Homemade natural laundry soap

1 bar (130g/4½oz) natural soap (like Dr. Bronner's Mild Aloe Baby Soap Bar)

1 cup of washing soda (like soda crystals)

Grate the soap in a food processor until finely ground. Once grated add in the washing soda. Blend the mixture together to create a powder. Store in a sealed container and use around ¼ cup per load of laundry.

Bath time

There are few experiences that relax and settle a baby quite like a bath. Bath time can establish a good bedtime pattern, which is key to ensuring that your child develops good sleeping habits, as children greatly benefit from the reassurance of regular activities and attention. Put simply, they love to know what's coming next!

Bath time can increase the bond between you and your baby, and helps to trigger oxytocin, which we like to call the cuddle hormone. After bathing dry your baby carefully, patting (not rubbing) with a soft towel. This is to protect the delicate skin cells, which are much thinner than an adult's. Check folds of skin to make sure that they are dry too, so that your baby's skin doesn't become sore or irritated. After drying apply a good additive-free baby moisturizer to keep the skin baby-soft.

Sam: "Make sure you have everything you need for bath time – a warm, comfortable towel, changing mat, organic bath wash – so you don't have to leave the bathroom. It's all about preparation."

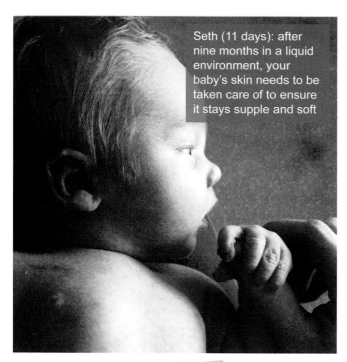

Seth (11 days): after nine months in a liquid environment, your baby's skin needs to be taken care of to ensure it stays supple and soft

Baby massage

If your baby suffers from minor skin complaints, massage can treat those issues too. Always use organic massage oils.

The ideal time is immediately after a lovely warm bath. There are so many benefits – well documented – to baby massage for both parent and child including bonding, reducing stress, aiding digestion and circulation, and giving your child the ability to self-soothe. It is a wonderful aid to calm fussy children, and can improve sleep patterns. (For directional bedtime baby massage, visit Mumma Love Organics' YouTube channel at: www.youtube.com/user/mummaloveorganics.)

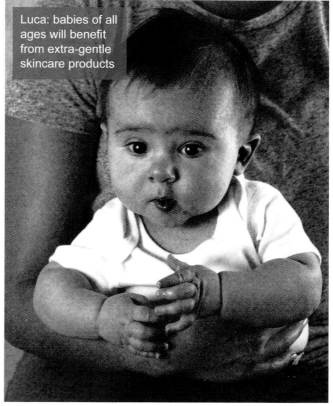

Luca: babies of all ages will benefit from extra-gentle skincare products

Homemade baby moisturizer

¼ cup of coconut oil
¼ cup of cocoa butter
1 tbsp beeswax
½ cup of sweet almond oil
Glass jar

In a pan gently melt the coconut oil, cocoa butter and beeswax, then add the sweet almond oil. Mix well, pour into a clean 115g (4oz) glass jar. Allow to cool. Use as you would a regular moisturizer for your baby. This recipe is great for babies with dry skin or eczema. It's also beneficial for stretchmarks!

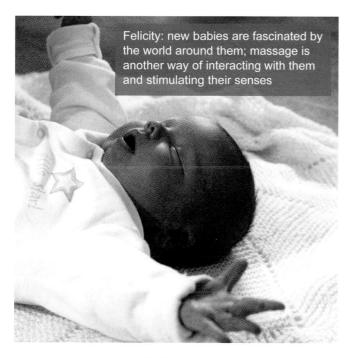

Felicity: new babies are fascinated by the world around them; massage is another way of interacting with them and stimulating their senses

Newborn skin complaints

If you are worried about your baby's skin, speak to your health visitor. That said, there is a range of common newborn skin complaints that your baby may suffer from in the first year of their life. These are likely to be one of the following:

- Baby eczema
- Dry skin
- Baby acne
- Cradle cap
- Nappy rash.

If you're breastfeeding, take a close look at your own diet to help eliminate foods that might be causing an issue for your baby's skin. The main foods that could cause your baby problems are cow's milk, peanuts, tree nuts (not peanuts, which are legumes) and shellfish.[6]

Here are some natural topical remedies to ease these skin complaints.

■ Baby eczema

Babies often get red, scaly skin known as eczema. Eczema – sometimes also known as dermatitis – is an inflammation of the skin that leads to redness, itching and flaking. Although there is no cure, there are many natural solutions to treat flare-ups.

Homemade bath recipe for eczema

For this recipe you will need a blender or food processor, and a cup of unflavoured oatmeal. (For young babies only half a cup.)

First, blend the oats on the highest setting to a fine powder.

To make sure it is the right consistency, stir 1 tbsp of oats into a glass of warm water: the water should turn milky, and the oats should easily absorb the water.

When the bath is running, sprinkle a small cup into the bath and stir so that the oatmeal is evenly distributed. If there are any large lumps at the bottom of the bath, break them up with your fingers.

Soak your child in the bath for 5 minutes and pat dry with a towel. Bear in mind that the bath will be more slippery than usual, so please take care.

■ Dry skin

A baby's skin is incredibly fragile. It is thin and easily dries out, which then leaves it susceptible to soreness, itching and red patches. This can happen when there are extremes of temperature including the weather, indoor heating and air conditioning. The chlorine from a swimming pool and salt water can also make a child's skin dry.

Baby-soft skin soap recipe

Soap mould

Sunflower oil

450g (16oz) water

225g (8oz) vegetable soap (grated and unscented)

30g (1oz) beeswax

30g (1oz) cocoa butter

1 tbsp coconut oil

1 tbsp oatmeal (finely ground)

1 tbsp honey (gently warmed)

Grease a soap mould with a little sunflower oil.

Heat the water until just before it boils and add the grated soap while stirring. Stir occasionally until melted and use a blender (with a little extra water) until it has a smooth texture. Then pour back into the saucepan.

When the soap is melted, add the beeswax, cocoa butter and coconut oil, and stir over a low heat until everything is combined.

Remove from the heat and add the oatmeal, ensuring that you mix it thoroughly. Add the honey and mix well.

Pour the mixture into the mould and cover with greaseproof paper. Leave for around 24 hours to set.

Take it out of the mould and leave for another 24 hours wrapped in the greaseproof paper.

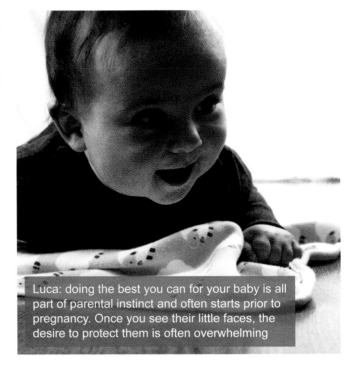

Luca: doing the best you can for your baby is all part of parental instinct and often starts prior to pregnancy. Once you see their little faces, the desire to protect them is often overwhelming

■ Baby acne

Baby acne, just like its teenage and adult counterparts, manifests as raised red bumps and spots on the skin. These can become worse when your baby is upset or tired, but it is not an especially serious issue — it usually clears up in its own time after the shared hormones between mother and baby dissipate. Acne is often more stressful for the parents.

Holly: "One of the most common conversations I've had with new parents is how quickly newborns shed their skin. After nine months in a completely different environment, things out here are going to be quite different. If your little one's skin is a little dry and flaky, then don't be alarmed, just keep it clean and soothe it with a natural remedy."

Homemade clear skin recipe

The age-old medicinal combination of honey and lemon isn't just for colds. Mix 1 tsp each of honey and lemon juice in a cup and, using a cotton bud, apply to the affected area. Keep away from the eyes and lips, and allow it to stay on the skin for at least 10 minutes. Next, using lukewarm water, use a sterile flannel to wipe the area you treated.

Calming cradle-cap recipe

1 tbsp raw shea butter
1 tbsp coconut oil
4 drops of organic lavender essential oil

Gently melt 1 tbsp of shea butter and 1 tbsp coconut oil in a pan till melted. Add 4 drops of lavender essential oil, mix well. Pour into a glass container, and use when required.

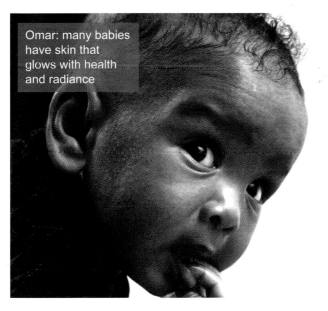

Omar: many babies have skin that glows with health and radiance

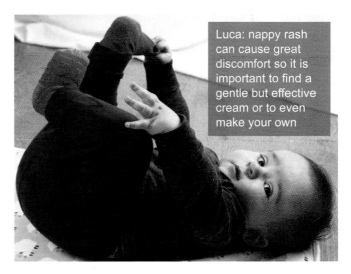

Luca: nappy rash can cause great discomfort so it is important to find a gentle but effective cream or to even make your own

■ Cradle cap

No one knows exactly why cradle cap appears, but these yellow, greasy-looking scaly patches on the scalp are very common. It can look alarming when the scabs begin to flake off and hair also comes away, but treating it early with organic solutions can help. It's important not to pick at the scales as this can cause an infection.[7]

■ Nappy rash

Nappy rash is redness and soreness on those areas usually covered by a nappy and occurs when skin has been in contact with ammonia (found in urine and poo). It can leave your baby in great discomfort.

Prevention is always best when it comes to nappy rash. This means changing your baby's nappy more often than you usually would. Cloth nappies can be kinder to the skin than standard disposable ones as they don't contain chemicals to aid absorption. Not only that, but cloth nappies are better for the environment (around 8 million disposable nappies are thrown away every day and it takes one disposable nappy 550 years to break down[8]) and your pocket in the long run. However, cloth nappies don't tend to absorb as much, so you will probably need to change more often. Consider investing in some partially biodegradable disposable nappies when you are on the move.

Natural nappy-rash cream

The ingredients are healing as well as soothing, and lavender oil, coconut oil and honey are all antibacterial. Altogether, this blend makes the perfect rash cream.

¼ cup of spring water	3 tbsp raw coconut oil
2 tbsp calendula flowers	5 drops of lavender essential oil
1 tbsp raw shea butter	5 drops of chamomile essential oil
1 tbsp raw cocoa butter	
1 tbsp beeswax	Glass jar

Mix the cup spring water with the calendula flowers. Simmer gently for 10-15 minutes. Strain, reserving the water.

In a separate pan gently melt the raw shea butter, cocoa butter, beeswax and coconut oil. Add 2 tbsp of the herbal liquid. Stir all together until everything is completely melted. Add the essential oils.

Pour into a very clean glass jar. Allow to cool, then use like normal nappy balm.

Suncare

Newborn babies are not designed to be exposed to strong sunlight, so try to keep your baby as shaded as possible for at least the first six months of their life. During this time, most sun protection creams are not suitable. Choose a lotion or spray made specifically for babies, which means it has been specially formulated to use on babies from 6 months of age. If your baby is younger than 6 months, it's best to keep them out of the sun altogether.[9]

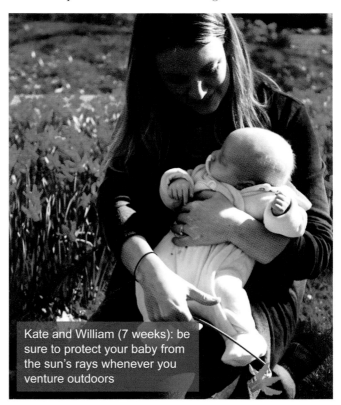

Kate and William (7 weeks): be sure to protect your baby from the sun's rays whenever you venture outdoors

Sam: "I have researched the healing powers of many natural ingredients over the years. One of my favourites is my nappy rash balm, which works a treat."

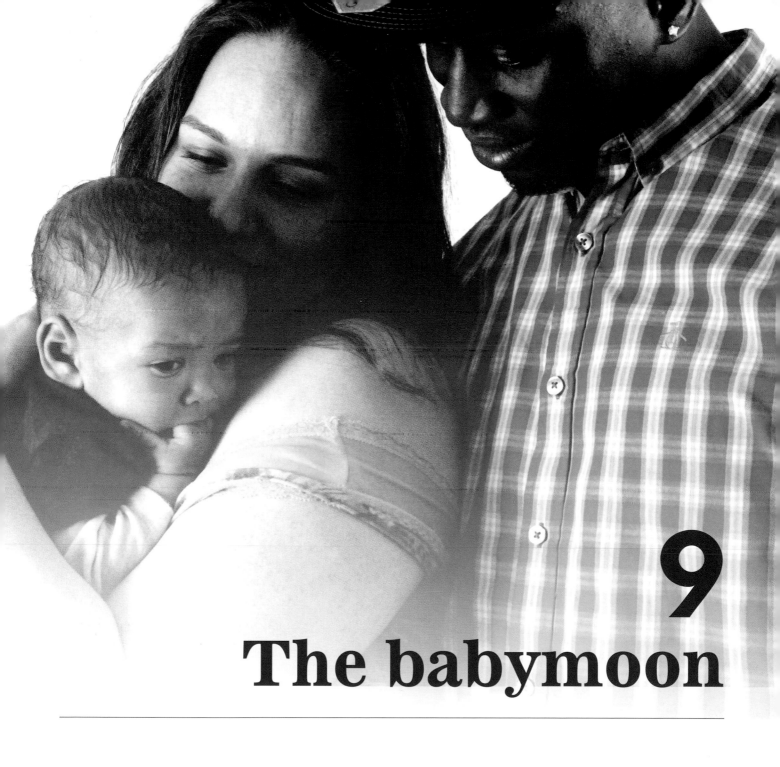

The babymoon

9

9
The babymoon

A babymoon is sometimes used to describe a final holiday taken by the couple prior to their baby's birth. It also refers to the practice of nesting: a period of around six weeks following the birth when the mother and her family are bonding with the baby. It is also when the mother is taken care of by family or friends. The focus is on relaxation and resting.

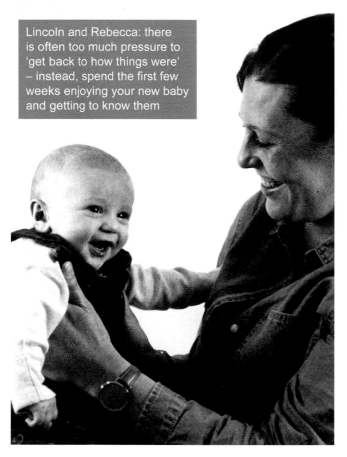

Lincoln and Rebecca: there is often too much pressure to 'get back to how things were' – instead, spend the first few weeks enjoying your new baby and getting to know them

This kind of babymoon is not normally practised in Western societies, but in Asian, Latin, Middle Eastern and indigenous cultures it is often the norm. Although the length of the postpartum period varies, the notion of a 40-day postpartum confinement is common in many non-Western cultures.[1] A number of ancient customs suggest that this is a necessity for new mothers, and is important in allowing her to adjust to the newness of motherhood. Therefore, it is also beneficial to the baby.

Pregnancy and birth are physically demanding, and the babymoon should ideally be used as a period of recuperation before the job of mothering gets fully underway. It seems the most sensible and natural thing in the world, so why is it not done more often in Western cultures? Why are women expected to carry on with their lives as if nothing world-changing has happened to them?

If we have major surgery, we are advised to rest for six weeks. Six weeks is the optimum time for a body to heal, and the same is true after a birth. Resting after giving birth gives the body the chance to recover more fully, so that those trips out – such as to the supermarket – which can seem utterly overwhelming if recovery is not complete, become much easier to handle.

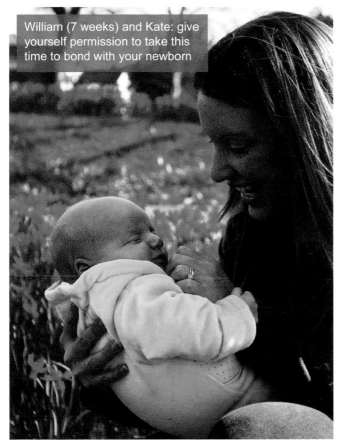

William (7 weeks) and Kate: give yourself permission to take this time to bond with your newborn

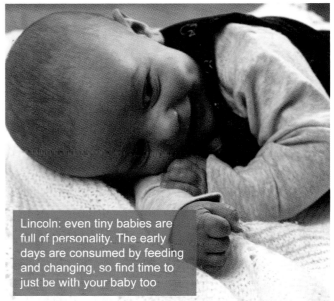

Lincoln: even tiny babies are full of personality. The early days are consumed by feeding and changing, so find time to just be with your baby too

We should respect our bodies, and rushing to get on with other jobs that can wait is doing no one any favours; you need to be healthy so that you can care for your baby. However, a babymoon might not run so smoothly if you have a toddler in tow. If you have other children, plan your babymoon realistically. You might not be able to relax to the fullest extent, but no one expects you to be on the school

Sam: "When I had my third child my midwife suggested that I stay in with him for a few weeks. This sounded strange to me especially since he was not my first baby, and no one else had mentioned such a thing to me before, but I soon understood that this was my chance to recover, and was as much for my well-being as my baby's. When I allowed myself this time, I not only healed well, but I had more energy. By just keeping the world at bay for a few weeks I was a much better mother."

run or doing the weekly shop days after giving birth. See if your partner can take extra paternity leave or save up his holiday to allow you time to rest. If you're a single parent, give yourself a break from the day-to-day housework chores or just focus on cooking quick and easy meals. The most important thing is that you rest and recover as much as you can without feeling guilty and under pressure from yourself. Resist the urge to be super-mum!

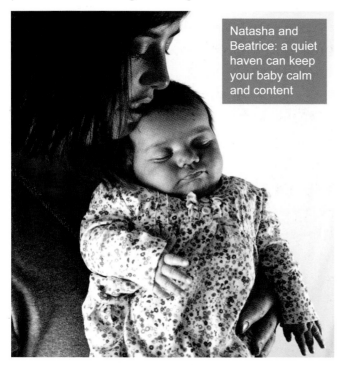

Natasha and Beatrice: a quiet haven can keep your baby calm and content

Create a safe, quiet haven

The best way to ensure your babymoon starts well is not to assume that you need to be up and about straight away. Follow your instincts and make a cosy, restful space for you and your baby at home, allowing you time to connect and bond. This might be in your bedroom or in your living room, perhaps both.

Trust your instincts

Many people feel under pressure to show off their new baby to their colleagues. Don't do anything you don't feel comfortable with. There will be time enough in the future, six months down the line or later, when you will have more of a handle on being a parent. Feel free to make your excuses. A mother has many instincts when it comes to her child, and it is when we listen to these instincts that a happier bonding experience can come about.

You may feel a commitment to take your baby out and show them to the world, but friends and family should understand if you choose not to do this for a while. You may want to discuss this before the birth so they know that you want a little time to yourself for the first few weeks. This will prevent any well-meaning phone calls or visitors landing on you unannounced before you are ready. However, immediate family are unlikely to want to wait for weeks to meet the baby, so why not set a date aside for short visits? Sometimes a babymoon will be enhanced by certain people.

Establishing the parameters of your babymoon means you can relax, knowing that you can truly enjoy this precious time without guilt.

Attachment parenting

Attachment parenting is a gentle shift away from the traditional model of the authoritarian parent to more of a one on connection. The aim is to raise secure children by listening to their needs and doing all you can to promote

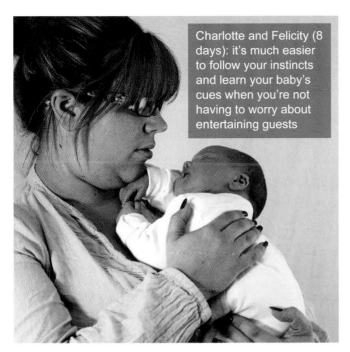

Charlotte and Felicity (8 days): it's much easier to follow your instincts and learn your baby's cues when you're not having to worry about entertaining guests

The babymoon is an important time to learn how to communicate with your baby. All the new feelings and emotions that a new baby feels can be overwhelming for them, no matter whether they are happy or sad. So reassurance from a parent or parents is crucial – but until a parent knows how to read their baby's emotions, it can be difficult to help. This settling-in time is ideal for learning as much as possible about your newborn, including how to read your baby's cues and how to respond to them.

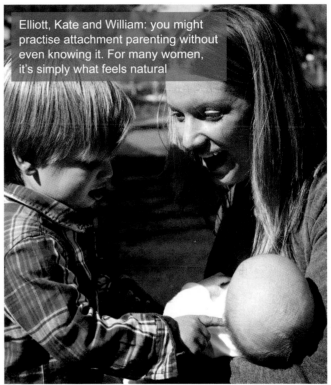

Elliott, Kate and William: you might practise attachment parenting without even knowing it. For many women, it's simply what feels natural

a secure and nurturing bond with your child. We believe that attachment parenting practices like baby-wearing, co-sleeping and responding to tantrums with sensitivity are what children need to thrive.

A person who, as a child, has had a secure attachment to their parent(s) is generally able to respond to stress in healthy ways and establish more meaningful and close relationships more often.[2] Babies are happiest when in close contact with their primary carer as this builds a foundation of trust at the beginning of infancy. Attachment parenting helps a parent to tune into what their child is communicating, helping them to respond consistently and appropriately. Babies cannot be expected to self-soothe and need calm, loving and empathetic parents to help them learn to regulate their emotions.[3] At this young age, they don't need much more than contact with their mother and milk. Attachment parenting is really about showering your baby with love and responding to their needs (it's that simple).

Attachment-parenting practices

Attachment parenting can be done in a way that suits you and your child, and no two ways will be the same.

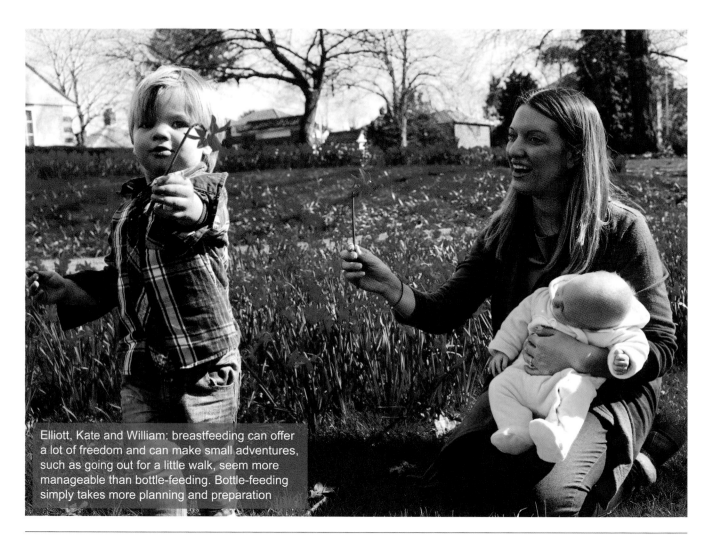

Elliott, Kate and William: breastfeeding can offer a lot of freedom and can make small adventures, such as going out for a little walk, seem more manageable than bottle-feeding. Bottle-feeding simply takes more planning and preparation

Holly: "When my daughter was a newborn I breastfed on demand, wore her in a papoose and co-slept at times, unaware that I was practising attachment parenting. Nowadays women can find communities of like-minded mums on the internet, and you can guarantee that some other poor sleep-deprived mum will be online at 3am while feeding on demand."

■ Breastfeeding

Not only are you giving them all the nutrients they need to grow healthy and strong, but the skin-to-skin contact is excellent at reinforcing your closeness. Breastfeeding also enables your body to produce the 'mothering hormone' prolactin, as well as oxytocin.

■ Baby-wearing

The first three months of a baby's life are known as the 'fourth trimester' since your baby will need so much help in the outside world. If it is possible to recreate the conditions of the womb, this will help to calm them immensely. Babies who are in close contact with their parents have been shown to have a higher level of oxytocin than non-carried babies, which subsequently helps to reduce stress in infants.[4]

Baby-wearing – carrying your baby in a sling or carrier – is not just for practicality (although it does free up your hands). It is also about keeping your baby close, and giving them the confidence that you will be there for them. A seminal 1986 study showed that babies of 6 weeks who received extra carrying cried and fussed 43 per cent less overall.[5]

Colic, reflux and wind can be alleviated if a baby is being held upright in a baby carrier, and their gross motor skills (eg, rolling over and sitting) won't be held back. In fact, because they become tuned in to their parent, they are more likely to be able to regulate their own movements quicker. This is because carried babies have more environmental experiences. These stimulate nerves to branch out and connect with other nerves, which helps the baby's brain to grow and develop.[6]

Oddly enough, ear infections can also be prevented through baby-wearing, and so can high or low temperatures. When babies are carried their respiratory rate, heart rate and body temperature are more stable.[7] The mother's body compensates for the baby's temperature, warming up if the baby is too cold, and cooling down if the baby is too hot. This is known as 'thermal synchronicity'.[8]

Studies have even shown that carried babies are able to develop new skills more quickly, including speaking and general communication skills. This is because carried babies spend more time in a state of quiet alertness, which may be called the most optimal state for learning.[9]

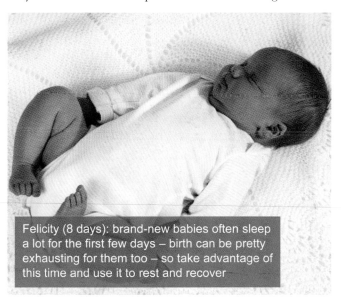

Felicity (8 days): brand-new babies often sleep a lot for the first few days – birth can be pretty exhausting for them too – so take advantage of this time and use it to rest and recover

■ Co-sleeping

Co-sleeping is often not a conscious decision, but more of a natural progression that happens after the baby is born, especially if the mother is breastfeeding. It is often much easier to feed and comfort your baby if you are in the same bed. Co-sleeping has happened for many centuries, and it is entirely natural. However, NICE (the UK's National Institute for Health and Care Excellence) acknowledge that there is an association between co-sleeping and Sudden Infant Death Syndrome (SIDS), especially if the baby has a low birth weight, and recommend that babies of 6 months and under sleep in a cot in their parents' bedroom.[10] Although most parents don't plan to sleep with their baby, around half of all mums in the UK do so at some time in the first few months after birth.[11] Many parents find that bringing their baby into their bed helps them to care for their baby at night. One Australian study found that 80 per cent of babies spent some time co-sleeping in the first six months of life.[12] With good careful planning there is no reason why co-sleeping can't be joyous and safe.

If you feel uncomfortable sleeping with your baby, there are a number of excellent sleeper cribs that attach to the side of the bed. This is a great compromise if your partner is not keen on sharing the bed with your child.

Co-sleeping means that a parent can be so much more responsive to their baby's needs, settling them more quickly before they can work themselves up into a frenzy. Co-sleeping is an excellent way to breastfeed on demand, which in turn regulates the breast milk supply.

Top tips for co-sleeping[13]

- The mattress must be firm to avoid overheating or suffocation
- Don't place the baby between you and your partner

- Use a lightweight cover for you and the baby or a baby sleeping bag – never a duvet. Make sure the temperature in the bedroom isn't too high. Your mattress should fit snugly against the wall to ensure your baby can't fall out of the bed or become trapped between the mattress and wall
- Never leave your baby unattended
- Always put your baby to sleep on their back
- Babies don't need a pillow and should be kept away from parents' pillows
- Never risk falling asleep with your baby on a sofa or armchair. If you're feeling really tired and think you may fall asleep with your baby while feeding or cuddling them on a sofa or armchair, move to a bed
- Don't let your baby and toddler sleep next to each other in case the toddler rolls on to your baby.

Co-sleeping should not take place[14] if either you or your partner:

- Smoke
- Have drunk alcohol (even a small amount)
- Have taken any drugs (prescribed or otherwise)
- Are extremely tired or have a sleep disorder.

NICE recommend you should not co-sleep if your baby is 6 months old or less, was premature or had a low birth weight.[15]

Sam: "My partner was anxious that something might happen to the baby if we co-slept, so we bought a co-sleeping bedside cot instead. I could still feed on demand and get a good night's sleep and he could sleep peacefully without worrying."

Holly: "If your children sleep in your bed, it may mean you need to be a little creative with your sex life. I sometimes wonder how people who practise attachment parenting manage to have more than one child! I like the idea of children having their own personal space but also knowing that their parents are around if they need reassurance, no matter what time of night it is."

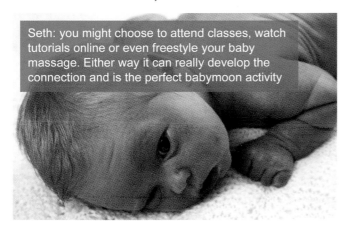

Seth: you might choose to attend classes, watch tutorials online or even freestyle your baby massage. Either way it can really develop the connection and is the perfect babymoon activity

Before committing to co-sleeping, make sure it is the route you and your partner want to take. If so, make a proper assessment of the sleeping area and make it absolutely safe for co-sleeping. If it is not safe enough, for example if you sleep in a double rather than a kingsize bed, then don't feel pressured into doing it; your childcare is your decision.

Some people worry that attachment parenting will make the baby clingy or too dependent, but the case is often completely the opposite; babies know that their parent will be there for them, no matter what, which gives them more confidence when they do have to go out on their own.

▪ Baby massage

Although newborns may not be able to see very well, their sense of touch is quite developed at birth. A gentle touch shows your child that you are there for them, physically and spiritually, and that they can trust you; this is why baby massage is so effective in nurturing your baby, and, if possible, should be part of your daily routine.

By scheduling a daily massage session, you can really ensure that the bond between you is strong. In a recent study, infants' sleep increased after massage, they were less restless and there was more mother–baby interaction.[16]

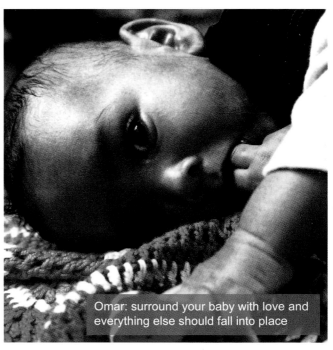

Omar: surround your baby with love and everything else should fall into place

Sam: "My first child was born prematurely and I still believe that baby massage saved her. At first she was too poorly to massage. I used to just lay my hands on her for comfort. This was less stimulating than patting or stroking, as she grew stronger I increased the massage strokes. I massaged her daily and watched her thrive. I still massage her to this day. I find it relaxes her when she's feeling down."

Humans as a species thrive on touch. Being held when we are sad or hurt, hugged when we are celebrating, even shaking hands on meeting someone new, gives us that reassuring contact we need. Babies are learning all the time, and they are soon able to distinguish between the different people who hold them, and they respond accordingly. Baby massage is a great way to indulge your child's need to be touched, while giving in to the parental instinct to show love and affection to their child.

You don't need to have gone on a specific massage course. There are baby massage classes available or plenty of videos online (see https://www.youtube.com/c/NaturalMumma).

Final thought

As long as you are loving, caring, calm and patient most of the time, you will become a successful parent, and your children will have every chance of becoming well-balanced, much-loved, happy healthy adults. (Remember that if you practise good self-care on a daily basis, whatever the degree of your caring commitments, you will find it easier to be loving, caring, calm and patient!)

Natural Dad: bonding with baby

Sometimes dads can feel a little lost during pregnancy, labour and birth. And once the baby has arrived, it can be even harder for partners to get a look in, especially when the baby is breastfeeding. Here are some tips on helping dad to bond with baby in the early days.

Play an active role in the pregnancy and birth

Lots of partners feel a little surplus to requirements during pregnancy and birth, but this time is when their support is needed more than ever. Studies have shown that a father's hormonal activity increases during pregnancy, and more so during birth (when a father spends a significant amount of time with his newborn, oxytocin encourages him to become more involved in the ongoing care of his child).[17] Skin-to-skin contact with dad is extremely beneficial for the bonding process and increases oxytocin production too. Remember, this is the hormone that is responsible for the nurturing instincts mums and dads need in order to form loving bonds with their babies.

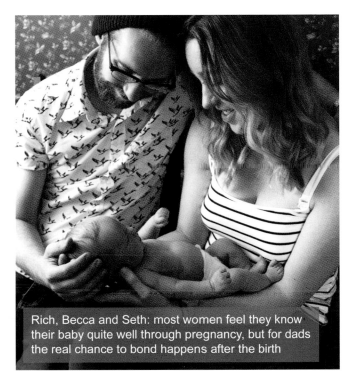

Rich, Becca and Seth: most women feel they know their baby quite well through pregnancy, but for dads the real chance to bond happens after the birth

Support your partner and baby's breastfeeding journey

A breastfeeding mother will spend the majority of her time with her baby, feeding, nurturing and nourishing on demand. And while this is essential both for her milk supply and for bonding with baby in the early weeks, it is also an extremely intense time. The relationship between mother and baby at this stage can feel a little isolating for partners, but there are ways that dad can make sure his bond with baby grows and develops too.

- Have patience. Mother and baby need time to establish breastfeeding and it might not be possible to help straight away. Be on hand to help whenever you are needed. Share in the night feeds wherever possible. Bring the baby to your partner for a feed, and try changing and winding the baby before and after feeds. Winding a baby is simple: place your baby over your shoulder with their bottom supported by your arm on that side. With your other hand, pat or rub their back. Alternatively, place the baby chest-down on your lap. Hold them firmly with one hand and pat or rub their back gently with the other.[18]

- Discuss the possibility of expressing breast milk into a bottle so that some feeds can be shared. Many women may not want to bottle-feed straight away, and it is recommended that breastfeeding is established before expressing, but it is an option worth considering when your baby is a little older.

- Praise your partner as she and baby learn how to develop their breastfeeding relationship. It's not always easy and the early days with a newborn can be overwhelming and exhausting. Be mindful of this, and make sure you let your partner know how fantastically well she is doing.

- Do as much housework as you can, so that your partner can focus on nurturing your baby without the distraction of too many household chores.

The early days may be full-on, but they don't last forever!

Holly: "A breastfeeding mother often starts her day with a feed. Breastfeeding on an empty stomach can make you feel quite dizzy, so breakfast in bed for the first few weeks at least would be very welcome."

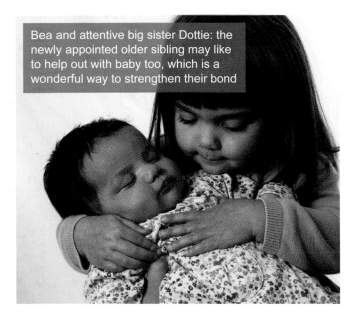

Bea and attentive big sister Dottie: the newly appointed older sibling may like to help out with baby too, which is a wonderful way to strengthen their bond

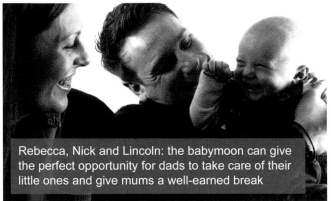

Rebecca, Nick and Lincoln: the babymoon can give the perfect opportunity for dads to take care of their little ones and give mums a well-earned break

Wear your baby close

There is no reason why dads can't wear their baby close too. Grab a sling or carrier and get bonding.

Make baby massage part of your daily routine

Baby massage helps to strengthen the bond between parent and child and is a wonderful way for dad to get involved. Baby and parent benefit from better and more relaxed sleep too.

Read to your baby

Studies have shown that it is usually mothers who take the time to read to their babies. You can change this! Spending time reading a book to your baby is a wonderful way to nurture a close and loving relationship and you'll be developing essential communication skills too.

Get stuck in

Change as many nappies as you can. Comfort your baby when they cry. Make sure that your voice soothes and calms them. The bond that you form is so important, and it's up to you to make sure it happens. Be as hands on as you can, and enjoy every precious moment.

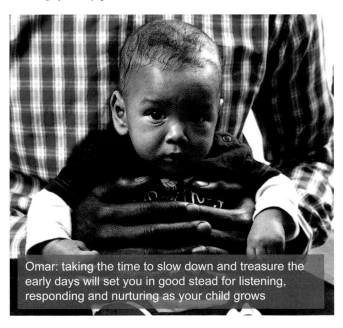

Omar: taking the time to slow down and treasure the early days will set you in good stead for listening, responding and nurturing as your child grows

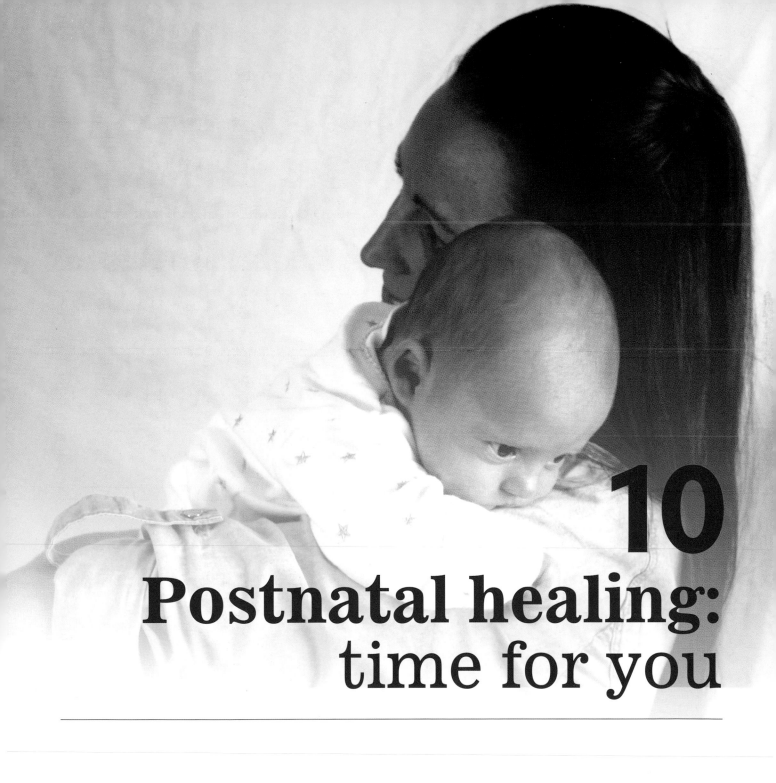

10

Postnatal healing:
time for you

10
Postnatal healing: time for you

Having a baby is one of the most life-changing experiences that a woman can go through. For nine months you have cherished the baby growing inside of you by adapting your diet, your lifestyle and your mindset to allow for the new life within your body. During birth, you are put through an incredible strain and no matter how your baby is delivered, the act of childbirth is a huge event that can leave your body feeling the after-effects deeply.

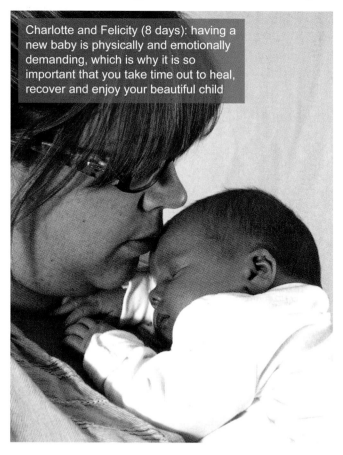

Charlotte and Felicity (8 days): having a new baby is physically and emotionally demanding, which is why it is so important that you take time out to heal, recover and enjoy your beautiful child

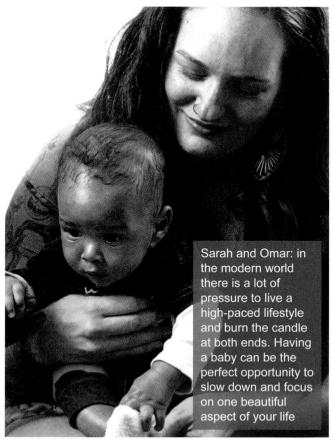

Sarah and Omar: in the modern world there is a lot of pressure to live a high-paced lifestyle and burn the candle at both ends. Having a baby can be the perfect opportunity to slow down and focus on one beautiful aspect of your life

It is not only your body that bears the hallmarks of pregnancy and birth. For many women, emotions can become jumbled and it can be hard to find yourself after such a major event, especially when you have a beautiful demanding newborn baby to take care of! It's not unusual to experience negative feelings towards your partner and even your baby after birth. Your hormones are a big player in this, so try not to worry; these symptoms will calm down. However, if you feel extremely low for a long period of time it's worth having a chat with your midwife as it could be postnatal depression. It's important to try to take care of yourself to limit these negative emotions. Here are some natural self-care tips to help.

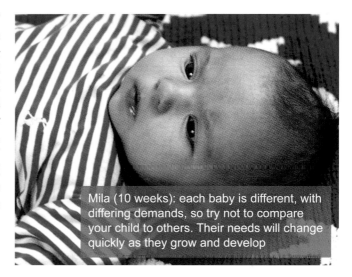

Mila (10 weeks): each baby is different, with differing demands, so try not to compare your child to others. Their needs will change quickly as they grow and develop

Accept your limitations

Mother nature rarely gives us more than we're able to manage, at least not in the short-term, but that doesn't mean you need to prove your ability to cope with it all by going above and beyond what is sensible. Pregnancy and birth are huge challenges for the body, and you aren't going to walk away from it all without a scratch. Chances are you will be very tired after your baby is born, so it's a good idea to take this as a signal to slow down and enjoy your babymoon.

Parenting a newborn involves round the clock care for a tiny person who is unable to fend for themselves. You're going to be required to do this straight after giving birth! So you're also going to need to accept that you can't do it all. Take this time to focus on your baby and your baby alone. Ask your partner to do the chores, or friends and family if you are fortunate enough to have a support network, and take everything one step at a time. If it is just you, don't worry too much about the housework and just focus on the essentials.

Give yourself time

First, you are you. You are not Mrs X from down the road (who always dresses like she's going for a job interview), nor are you celebrity Y from Hollywood (who has a team of nannies away from the paparazzi's cameras). It doesn't matter how other mothers are seemingly coping with the pressures of parenthood; what matters is how you are feeling. Don't pile unnecessary pressure on yourself to perform miracles in the form of a supermarket run two days after the birth, or loads of washing and drying the minute you are home with your bundle of joy. You need to rest. You need to spend quality time with your baby.

Experts estimate that it can take a good six weeks to physically recover from giving birth,[1] but it's important to remember that this is just an estimate. If you need longer, be kind to yourself. Life doesn't have to be a race, and if you slow the pace a little you and your baby will benefit. So if help is offered, take it with both hands and enjoy this special time while you can. View pregnancy and birth as a slow marathon and give yourself a chance to catch your breath.

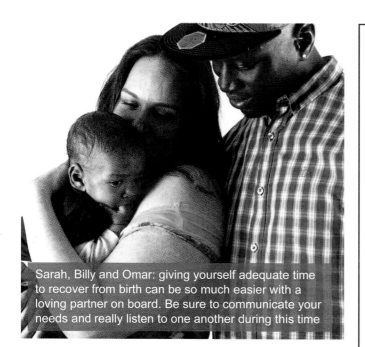

Sarah, Billy and Omar: giving yourself adequate time to recover from birth can be so much easier with a loving partner on board. Be sure to communicate your needs and really listen to one another during this time

Ask for help

Not everyone will realize how exhausting being a new mother can be (even other mothers often forget what it was like, particularly if they managed to bounce back after birth) so you may need to ask for help. If this is difficult for you, ask your partner to step in. Witness the famous proverb that 'It takes a village to raise a child'.

Around one in six mothers suffer from postnatal depression, although it's not always diagnosed.

Symptoms of postnatal depression

- Feeling very low or viewing life as a long, grey tunnel without end or hope
- Extreme tiredness or lethargy, or sometimes feeling numb, not wanting to do anything or take an interest in the outside world
- A sense of inadequacy, feeling unable to cope
- Feeling guilty about not coping or about not loving your baby enough
- Excessive irritability
- Being tearful and crying a lot
- Difficulty sleeping: either not getting to sleep or waking through the night (on your own accord)
- Having panic attacks
- Regular nightmares and irrational thoughts
- Overpowering anxiety often about issues that wouldn't normally bother you, such as being in the house on your own
- Regular difficulty in concentrating
- Physical symptoms: stomach cramps, headaches and blurred vision
- Obsessive fears that something might happen to your baby.

Sam: "After my second child I tried to be super-mum but came back down to reality with a crash. I made a conscious decision with my third to slow down and just be in the moment. I recovered quicker and as a result was a much better mum to all my kids."

Holly: "I put a lot of pressure on myself. As well as doing all I could for my baby, I also felt like I should be losing weight quickly, looking good and keeping the house sparkling. Give yourself the permission to just cope with raising the miracle that your baby is. Let the dishes pile up a little and don't strive for perfection. It is love and compassion that make women beautiful, not tiny figures and time to do their make-up. Keep your hair wild and your heart open; these baby days fly past, so cherish each moment."

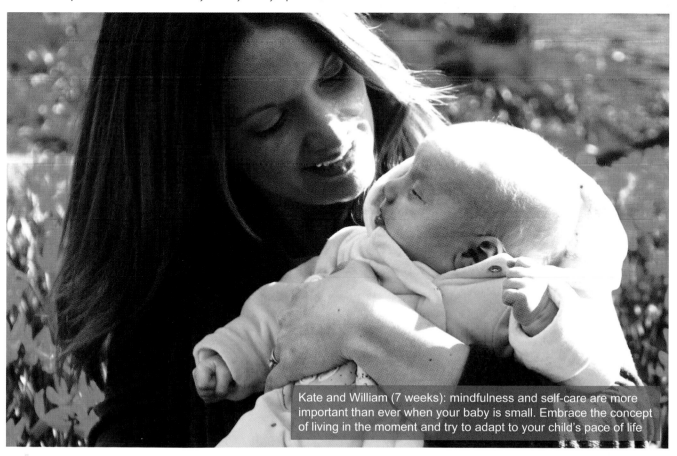

Kate and William (7 weeks): mindfulness and self-care are more important than ever when your baby is small. Embrace the concept of living in the moment and try to adapt to your child's pace of life

If you are suffering from some of these symptoms, talk to someone. You are going through a huge transitional stage in your life. A sympathetic listener, who will enable you to express your feelings and worries without fear of judgement, can bring enormous relief. This may be your health visitor or partner, your community midwife, counsellor or friend. Please don't suffer in silence.

Talk

If you are feeling upset, emotional or confused about how you're coping, or about how well you think your baby (or your partner) is doing, don't keep emotions bottled up. Your partner, friends, family and health visitor are all there to listen to you and help you if it's needed. Lots of women find the early days of parenthood extremely difficult and there is nothing to be ashamed of in reaching out.

Eat well

Not only do you need extra energy to cope with the demands of a new baby, especially if you are breastfeeding, but what you eat can directly affect your mood. Try to include as many nutrients as possible in each meal and snack. Foods such as:

- Dark leafy greens
- Root vegetables
- Fresh fruit
- Avocados
- Coconut

are all great for helping to boost your system after birth. Try to avoid processed foods, refined sugars and alcohol, however tempting these shortcuts may be.

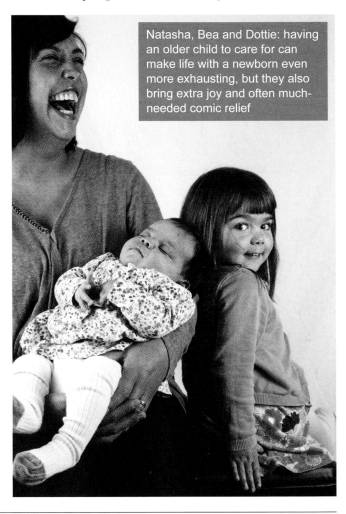

Natasha, Bea and Dottie: having an older child to care for can make life with a newborn even more exhausting, but they also bring extra joy and often much-needed comic relief

Holly: "The healthier you are and more balanced you feel, the more energy and patience you will have for your family. Sometimes all it takes is permission from yourself."

Exercise

Depending on when you feel able, or when your doctor deems you ready, take on some gentle exercise to help boost serotonin levels in the body. The release of serotonin helps to reduce stress, aid appetite, ward off depression and improve your mood. Start by taking walks with the pram. And don't push yourself too hard – pace yourself and enjoy the fresh air for a while. Try walking in your local park, or in local woodland. After your six-week check you can start a simple yoga routine to boost your energy (let your instructor know you've just had a baby, especially if you have had a c-section).

Elliott, William and Kate: keeping active is an important part of your physical and mental well-being. A gentle stroll in the park can make all the difference to the whole family

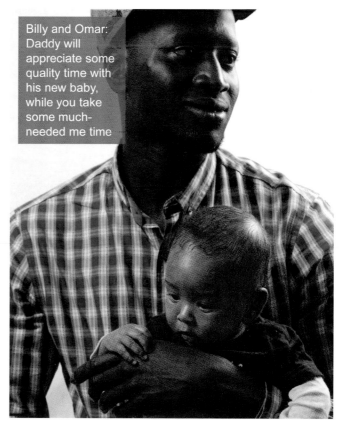

Billy and Omar: Daddy will appreciate some quality time with his new baby, while you take some much-needed me time

Make time for yourself

It's easy to forget what you enjoy doing after you've had a baby. The little things that used to make you happy like taking a long bath with a good book, walking in nature with your headphones on, for example, may not be possible now. This is why it is important to grab those precious minutes when your baby is sleeping and your other children, if you have them, are occupied. Here are some tips:

- Take that bubble bath! Pour a few drops of lavender oil into the water and relax

- Take a walk in the woods. Yes, it still can be done! Just invest in a good wrap or baby carrier

- Listen to music. Even if you are not able to walk in the woods at the same time, it doesn't mean your ears have to miss out.

Postnatal bath soak

¼ cup of calendula flowers
    (reduces inflammation and soothes irritated skin)

½ cup of lavender flowers
    (antiseptic and anti-inflammatory)

2 cups of water

¼ cup of yarrow flowers (anti-inflammatory)

¼ cup of Epsom salt (healing)

Mix flowers together and boil in water. Allow to cool before straining. Once strained add the Epsom salt. Put in your bath and enjoy a nice soak for around 20 minutes.

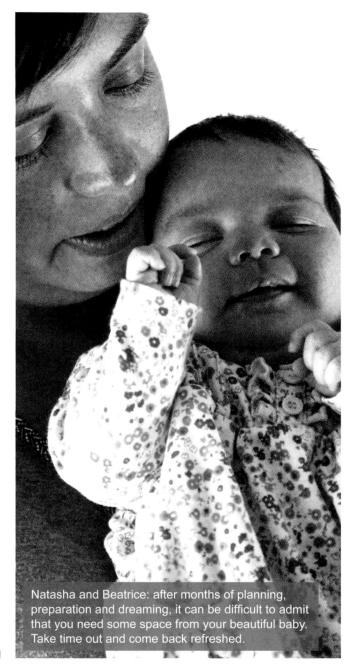

Natasha and Beatrice: after months of planning, preparation and dreaming, it can be difficult to admit that you need some space from your beautiful baby. Take time out and come back refreshed.

Natural Dad
Dads need nurturing too

New research has found that 38 per cent of dads are concerned about their own mental health.[2] It is normal to feel a little left out after all the anticipation of pregnancy and birth, especially if your partner is breastfeeding. Sleep deprivation doesn't help either. So how can we nurture dads a little more, and ensure that they are able to fully support their partner and enjoy life with their newborn baby?

Strive to find a new routine

Sometimes it helps dads to feel more involved if they are able to take on different responsibilities within the family: maybe doing the grocery shop, preparing the baby's bath at the end of the day, trying baby massage or giving the occasional bottle. Finding a new routine can help dads to begin the bonding process too.

Prepare for the sleepless nights

Sleep deprivation is challenging and it can play havoc with your emotions whether you're chock-full of postnatal hormones or not. And for dads, returning to work on very

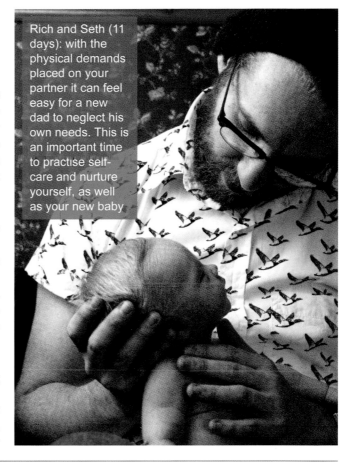

Rich and Seth (11 days): with the physical demands placed on your partner it can feel easy for a new dad to neglect his own needs. This is an important time to practise self-care and nurture yourself, as well as your new baby

Holly: "We thought that having a baby would fit in easily with our life. We might not be able to go to the cinema for a few months, but on the whole it shouldn't shake our world too much. Right? But when you actually have children, you are constantly on call. Even when they are at secondary school, they are firmly in the centre of your life. Nothing prepares you for how demanding it is to be a parent, but you're not prepared for how absolutely rewarding, joyful and fulfilling it is either."

little sleep can be really hard, especially when they are also striving to support their partners and take on extra duties at home. So go to bed earlier and clear the next few weekends of social commitments or DIY so that you can have some quality time doing very little. Take it in turns to sleep in.

Support your partner

Remember that she has been through a lot, and having a new baby to care for is going to take some getting used to. There are tasks that dads can take on such as emptying the dishwasher, putting clothes away and doing homework with any older kids. This will help the household to run more smoothly and your partner to recover more quickly.

Open up to your partner

Lots of dads feel that they are not supposed to talk about how they feel, but relationships are two-way streets, and it's important to acknowledge how both of you are feeling. Take the time to talk to each other.

Be kind to your partner

Take the time to regularly praise each other, and to appreciate what each of you brings to the family. Celebrate your achievements, no matter how small they may seem. And be kind to each other. Having a new baby is enormous, and not many of us come out the other side unscathed. But having a new baby is also one of the most amazing experiences you will have together, so enjoy this unique time and each other.

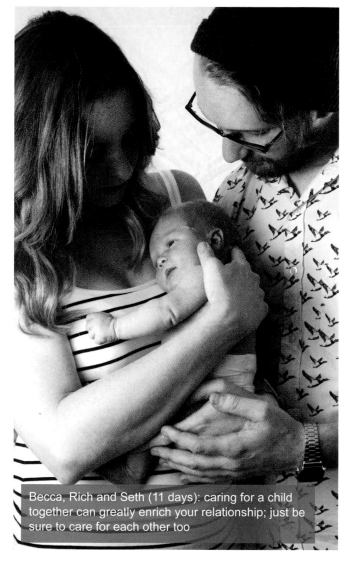

Becca, Rich and Seth (11 days): caring for a child together can greatly enrich your relationship; just be sure to care for each other too

Holly: "It can be especially hard for men to admit when they need help. This is something we can address when raising little boys. It's time we lost this notion to 'man up' and looked out for each other, regardless of gender."

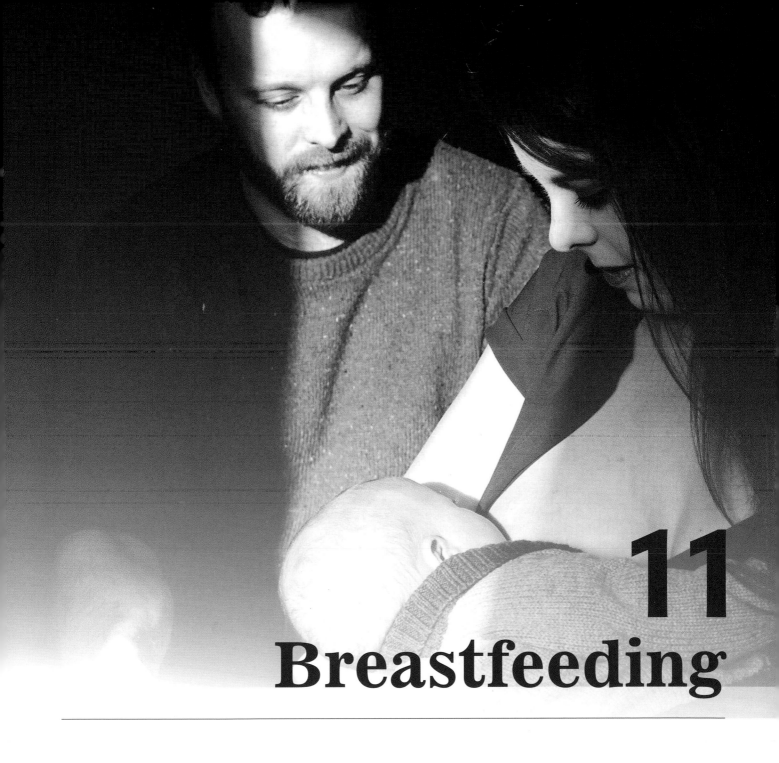

11
Breastfeeding

11
Breastfeeding

There are many things that new mums are faced with and breastfeeding can come with a whole host of questions, niggling worries and confusion. Here are a few handy tips to make things easier.

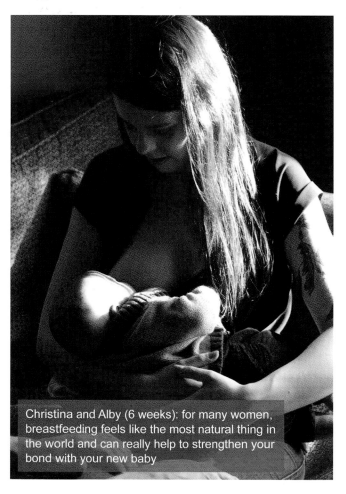

Christina and Alby (6 weeks): for many women, breastfeeding feels like the most natural thing in the world and can really help to strengthen your bond with your new baby

Value skin-to-skin

Skin-to-skin contact throughout the breastfeeding period will help your baby to breastfeed properly. If your partner wants to feed expressed milk to the baby, dads and babies may also find that skin-to-skin is the best approach.

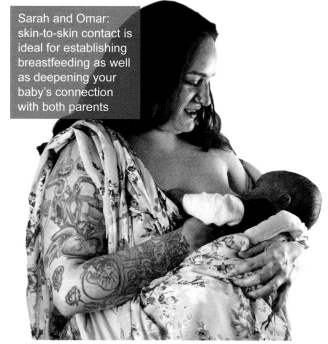

Sarah and Omar: skin-to-skin contact is ideal for establishing breastfeeding as well as deepening your baby's connection with both parents

Ride the first two weeks out

To begin with it's often hard to know if your baby is properly latched on. Even if they are, your nipples can feel sore. Many mums say that it took them a fortnight to develop this new skill and feel comfortable with breastfeeding.

Find support locally

Probably most new mothers are initially daunted by the idea of feeding in public and find it can restrict their routine. Finding a group of women in the same situation can be invaluable. Chat with your health visitor, Google local breastfeeding services and scour social media for support groups — or why not set up a local group yourself? Set up a social media page with advice and initiate discussions. Hire a hall and print posters, or ask a friendly local café if you can have a regular meet there. They'll benefit from sales of teas and coffees and you will all have a welcoming environment to relax and feed in.

Surveys show that the majority of people don't mind women breastfeeding in public at all — you should never be made to feel uncomfortable. In fact, the UK's Equality Act of 2010 made it illegal for anyone to ask a breastfeeding woman to leave a public place, such as a café, shop or public transport.[1] In Australia, women have the right to breastfeed anytime, anywhere. The Canadian Charter of Rights and Freedoms protects the rights of breastfeeding mothers to also feed anytime, anywhere. In New Zealand, there are no specific laws regarding breastfeeding — see New Zealand's Human Rights Commission for more information (https://www.hrc.co.nz/your-rights/social-equality/our-work/right-breastfeed/). In America, the laws vary from state to state. The first few times you may find breastfeeding in public a little strange, but as soon as you realize that no one is paying you any attention you'll soon be doing it without thinking.

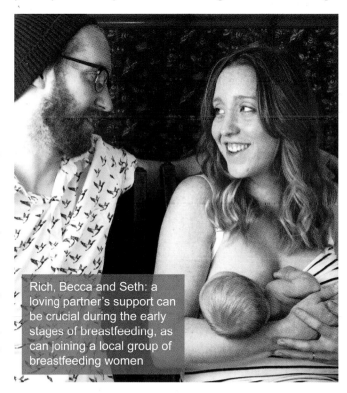

Rich, Becca and Seth: a loving partner's support can be crucial during the early stages of breastfeeding, as can joining a local group of breastfeeding women

Sam: "After my second child was born I joined a local breastfeeding support group. It was the right decision. Encouraged by these weekly meetings, I went on to feed Yasmin and Max till they were over a year old."

Don't take breastfeeding for granted

We all know about the benefits of breastfeeding, but it is really important not to judge women who are bottle-feeding. Many women would love to be able to breastfeed but are unable to do so. Give them an encouraging smile and feel blessed if you are able to breastfeed your child.

Follow your instincts

Have faith in your own natural maternal instincts and be led by your baby. The amount of time they feed for is bound to vary. As your child grows their nutritional needs will change, so if they need to feed more regularly or go for longer between feeds then don't panic. It is common for a newborn baby to need around 8-12 feeds a day, sometimes more. You can't overfeed a breastfed baby, so just be led by them. However, some babies will start to use the nipples as a comforter, so if your baby is sucking without taking any milk it would be worth making sure you only let them on the breast to feed. It can be easy to let your baby slip into the habit of falling asleep on the breast, especially when you are tired yourself. However, this is often the main reason why babies come to use their mum's nipples as a dummy / pacifier.

To stop this habit, make sure that your baby is always awake for their feed. A gentle tickle on the feet will usually stir them. If they are still rooting around looking for comfort, then gently applying pressure on their chin to shut their mouth can help them to self-soothe. After a feed, give your baby plenty of soothing cuddles to replace the comfort of the nipple. If they resist, it may be easier for the baby's dad to provide the comfort. This can be a hard cycle to break, but will help you to avoid the use of a dummy/pacifier and help your baby to learn to sleep by themselves. This should lead to restful nights for the whole family.

Don't be afraid to ask for help

Many women take to breastfeeding with ease while others really struggle. And just because you found it easy to feed your first child doesn't mean that things will be the same with subsequent children. Many hospitals offer postnatal classes in breastfeeding, and staff on the postnatal ward should also be on hand to offer advice. Chat to other mums; ask your health visitor, midwife and doctor.

Sam: "I stopped breastfeeding Ella shortly after she was born, a decision I later regretted, but at the time Ella wouldn't latch on properly and I was concerned about her weight. We both relaxed a little when I put her on the bottle. However, sometimes I felt judged. We all know breast is best, so there's usually a story behind a bottle-fed newborn."

Holly: "I wish someone had advised me when Jasmine was a baby not to let her fall asleep on the breast. Expecting me to be there when she woke and struggling to sleep without me meant that even after I stopped feeding her, she still woke several times a night for many years. Breaking this cycle during the early months would have meant that we all slept more soundly in later years. Dealing with sleep issues with an older child can be much more challenging, so finding strategies when your baby is small can be very helpful."

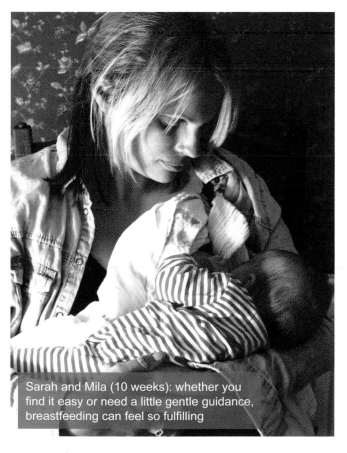

Sarah and Mila (10 weeks): whether you find it easy or need a little gentle guidance, breastfeeding can feel so fulfilling

There are a number of fantastic organizations that can offer you support, such as the Association of Breastfeeding Mothers, National Childbirth Trust (NCT) and the National Breastfeeding Helpline in the UK. In the USA, there are many groups including Wellstart International and Breastfeeding USA. The Australian Breastfeeding Association does great work in Australia and the New Zealand Breastfeeding Alliance is another such group. La Leche League exists in Canada and throughout the world. Your midwives, doctors or health visitors will be able to advise you what is on offer in your area.

Mark the side

Many women forget which side they last fed from. It may feel obvious as one breast may feel much fuller, but in a day when one feed blurs into the next it is easy to forget. Swapping a bracelet from wrist to wrist may help. It's not ideal for night feeds, but you can always change your child's position in the cot and use that as an indicator. If you last fed from the left breast, for example, then lay them down with their head at the other end of the cot so that next time you pick them up they are in the correct position to feed.

Lose the disposable nursing pads

Some women don't need pads. Those who do may find that disposables are too thin and can slip out during a feed. Washable breastpads are generally more durable and work out cheaper.

Consider a breastfeeding pillow

Pregnancy puts a massive strain on your back and pregnancy hormones loosen your ligaments.[2] It takes a while to get your back strong again when you are carrying a baby or a toddler. Exhaustion, lack of sleep and a decrease in core stability can lead to slumping during feeding, which can generate back pain and tension.

Breastfeeding pillows are specially made for optimum comfort for mother and baby and aim to enable you to place your child at the perfect position to latch on; they are also less likely to collapse so will avoid the need for further readjustment, which can be stressful for both of you. Whether or not you decide to invest in a special

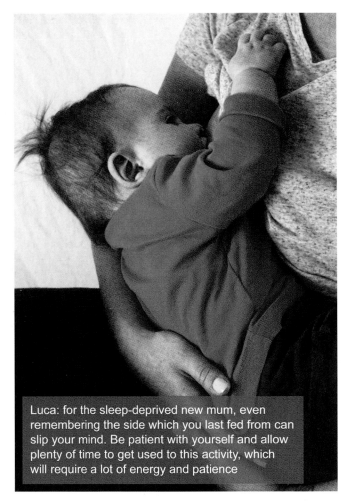

Luca: for the sleep-deprived new mum, even remembering the side which you last fed from can slip your mind. Be patient with yourself and allow plenty of time to get used to this activity, which will require a lot of energy and patience

Holly: "I had horrendous backache from the night feeds. During the day I was watching my posture but in the early hours I could barely keep my eyes open, let alone sit up properly. I started putting Jasmine in bed next to me and letting her feed as I lay down, which took so much pressure off my back (and meant I could snatch a few moments of extra sleep too!)."

breastfeeding pillow (try NCT sales if you are in the UK or eBay for secondhand options), be aware of your own posture while breastfeeding.

While sitting, you may need to lay several pillows under your child to achieve the right height. For night feeds, try lying on your side with your baby lying parallel to you.

Cracked nipples

Sore and cracked nipples can put an unhappy slant on breastfeeding, so it is much better to take care of your nipples from the off or at least be prepared in case they do get chapped. Breast milk itself has great healing properties so after each feed simply hand express a few drops of milk and smear them over the nipple area. Allow to dry naturally.

Otherwise, use organic natural oils. For example, coconut oil and olive oil are very nourishing and as they contain no chemicals are safe for your child. Calendula cream is very effective and safe too. You will also find that exposing your nipples to the air is very beneficial, so while breastfeeding at home spend as much time as possible without a top on!

Top tips for latching on

Problems with latching on are extremely common and can quickly lead to sore nipples. Bring your child to your breast and try to let them latch on by themselves rather than guiding them too much. This method may take a while to perfect, but is the best way to find the right position.

It can take up to two weeks for your nipples to acclimatize to being regularly suckled. But if breastfeeding feels painful, check with a professional and see if they can help you find a more comfortable position.

Top tips for successful breastfeeding

- Do your research: ask a breastfeeding friend If you can watch how her baby latches on; attend a breastfeeding class before the baby is born; read up on the subject (*The Food of Love* by Kate Evans, published by Myriad Editions, is particularly good)
- Reclining at a 45° angle can help you to relax and find a good position
- Start as soon as possible after your baby is born, ideally using skin-to-skin contact to help trigger the letdown reflex and relax you and the baby
- Squeeze a little milk out and rub it on your baby's bottom lip, and bring them close to the nipple. They will smell it and nuzzle closer, and will try to latch on by themselves
- Look for signs that your baby is properly latched on, such as a pulling sensation in the breast and movement in their jaw as they swallow. If this is not happening, the baby may not be getting any milk. Start again, trying a different position
- If it is incredibly painful, your baby may have not latched on properly, so try inserting a clean finger into their mouth to take them off the nipple and encourage them to try a different angle
- Give yourself and your baby time to learn this new skill. It might take perseverance for the first couple of weeks. Usually, following the baby's lead means that you will find a position that is most comfortable for you both.

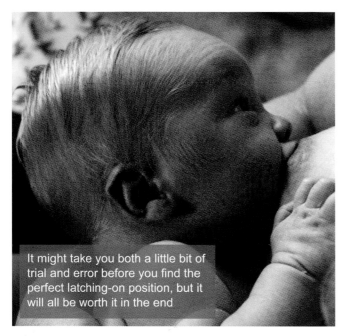

It might take you both a little bit of trial and error before you find the perfect latching-on position, but it will all be worth it in the end

Blocked milk ducts

Blocked milk ducts can lead to mastitis (inflammation of the mammary gland due to a bacterial infection). If your breasts do not seem to be draining, or your child seems unsatisfied with the feed, you may have a blocked duct. Check the breast area for a small knot or lump around the nipple. Try a hot shower, massage the area and try to hand express some milk to get things flowing again. Stay calm. Stress will make matters worse and a blocked milk duct is perfectly treatable.

Mix 2 drops of lavender essential oil with 1 tsp of coconut oil and massage into the entire breast area (right up into the armpit), then apply grated potatoes to the area and keep in place with a clean cloth or bra. Leave the potatoes in place for at least an hour. It sounds crazy, but this is a great way to unblock the duct! Chilling the potatoes first can be very effective as the coolness in the potatoes will reduce the heat from the inflammation. It is thought that the high starch in the potatoes draws out the infection. Traditionally, potatoes were used as a poultice for all manner of infections.

Sunflower lecithin is a great natural remedy to help thin the breast milk and make it less sticky. Take 1 x 1,200mg capsule 3-4 times a day. After a week or two without a blockage you can reduce the dosage by 1 capsule a day. Two weeks later reduce the dosage by another capsule. You may find that stopping the lecithin completely causes the blockage to return, in which case keep taking 1-2 capsules a day. There are no known contraindications for breastfeeding mothers using this natural remedy.

The best position for feeding once you have treated a blocked duct is from above as gravity will help with the milk flow. Gently lay your baby on a soft blanket on their back and feed using your elbow to support yourself.

Sometimes a blocked duct can be caused by ill-fitting bras. Your breasts will change a lot during pregnancy and after your baby is born. Ensuring that your bras fit can seem like a hassle, but it is really important to have a properly fitted bra, especially when breastfeeding.

Blocked ducts can be caused by stopping a feed before the breast is properly drained. It is so important never to rush feeds and to take as long as your baby needs.

Mastitis

Mastitis can be very painful, making feeding feel unbearable. Ideally, you want to feed during this time though or your breasts will become even more engorged. The age-old remedy of placing chilled cabbage leaves in the bra is a proven way to draw out the infection. Once the leaves start to wilt, replace them with fresh leaves from the fridge. You can compost the leaves.

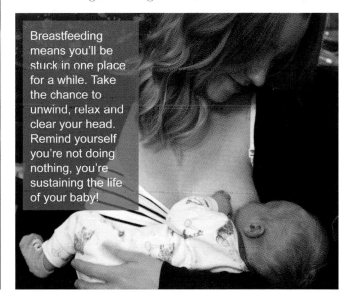

Becca and Seth: letting go of feeling any pressure to be perfect is the best approach to breastfeeding. It may be challenging to start with, but it is likely to become second nature

Using hot and cold compresses can help. The heat will open the milk ducts and draw out the infection while the cold will help the swelling to reduce. Using heat for 15-30 minutes prior to nursing can be really beneficial, and applying ice afterwards will help numb the pain.

It is vital to drink lots of water while breastfeeding to keep your fluid levels up, but it is even more important if you are fighting an infection such as mastitis. You also need to be sure to rest properly as many professionals believe that mastitis is a sign of being overtired.[3]

Breastfeeding means you'll be stuck in one place for a while. Take the chance to unwind, relax and clear your head. Remind yourself you're not doing nothing, you're sustaining the life of your baby!

Holly: "Mastitis was the reason I stopped feeding. I didn't know about the natural remedies and I became quite ill. If you do have to give up feeding earlier than expected, then please don't beat yourself up, but focus on the fact that you fed at all. The transition from breast to bottle can take some getting used to, and having to sterilize bottles and heat milk can seem quite inconvenient after breastfeeding, so give yourself time to adjust."

Nursing basket

It helps to have everything you need on hand when you are feeding as you are going to be staying put for a little while. Here are some suggestions:

- A bottle of water (staying hydrated is essential)
- Some dried fruit or an energy bar (breastfeeding burns off between 300 and 500 calories every day so keeping your nutrients up is vital)
- A manicure set? Filing your nails and hand lotion will help to pamper you
- A good book and some magazines
- A notebook, paper and pen (in case anything you need to remember pops into your head)
- Your iPod or music device
- A comfy blanket in case your little one gets cold
- A spare pair of baby socks
- A burp cloth
- Nipple cream or oil
- Your mobile phone.

Try putting a nursing basket in your bedroom and one in your living room.

Stay hydrated

Breast milk is around 90 per cent water.[4] Research shows that nursing mothers need around 3 litres (about 12 cups) of water a day, as opposed to the approximate 2 litres (8 cups) that the rest of us aim for in the ideal world. Try to pour yourself a drink of water with every feed.

Be prepared to put the time in

Breastfeeding cannot be rushed. Remember that you are doing a vital job, so don't give yourself a hard time if you don't feel like you are achieving much else. Feeding a child is a wonderful thing to be doing, and remember that breastfeeding burns a lot of calories. Take the time to relax, rest and bond with your beautiful baby.

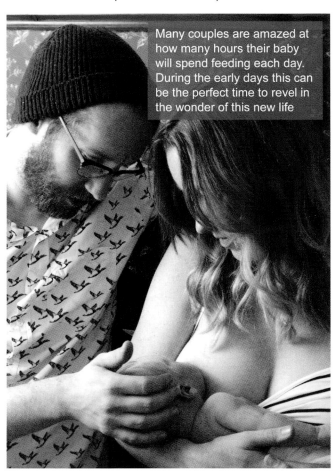

Many couples are amazed at how many hours their baby will spend feeding each day. During the early days this can be the perfect time to revel in the wonder of this new life

Wear the right clothes

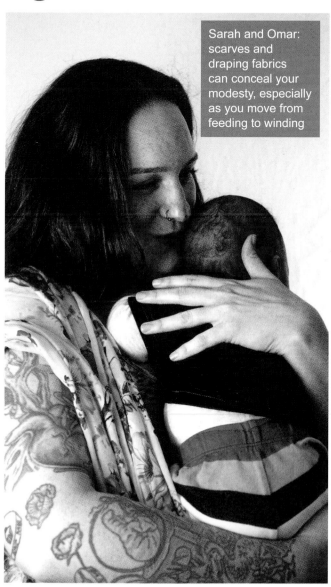

Sarah and Omar: scarves and draping fabrics can conceal your modesty, especially as you move from feeding to winding

Large scarves and pashminas are perfect for draping over a shoulder, to avoid exposing your breast. Deep V crossover tops that tie under the bust are beautifully flattering for new mums as well as allowing easy access to your boobs. Drape the scarf, unclip your nursing bra and bring your breast out and bring your baby to you. With a little practice this can be done without exposing any flesh at all. If you aren't a person who wears scarves, then a loose-fitting T-shirt can be perfect: wear it over a vest top and you can keep your baby concealed under the expansive T-shirt fabric. Try doing it in front of a mirror for a bit of reassurance, as you may well be surprised at how little is on show.

Make a list of perfect pit-stops

Breastfeeding is not illegal but if the idea of feeding in public is offputting, then be sure to compile a list of places that actively welcome breastfeeding. Some cafés and restaurants will display signs showing that they welcome nursing mothers. You may also find that some shops offer a comfortable place to stop and feed, especially large stores. Do your research before you leave home so that you will always feel confident about where you can breastfeed in the area that you are in.

Table service may work better, as trying to queue up with a hungry vocal baby and carry your drink with a pushchair may be too much to handle. It is also important to remember that for the few highly publicized negative comments that women have received for breastfeeding in public, there are millions who breastfeed every day without ever hearing a negative word. Many women who bottle-feed also feel judged. However you feed your baby be sure to remind yourself that you are doing the best you possibly can.

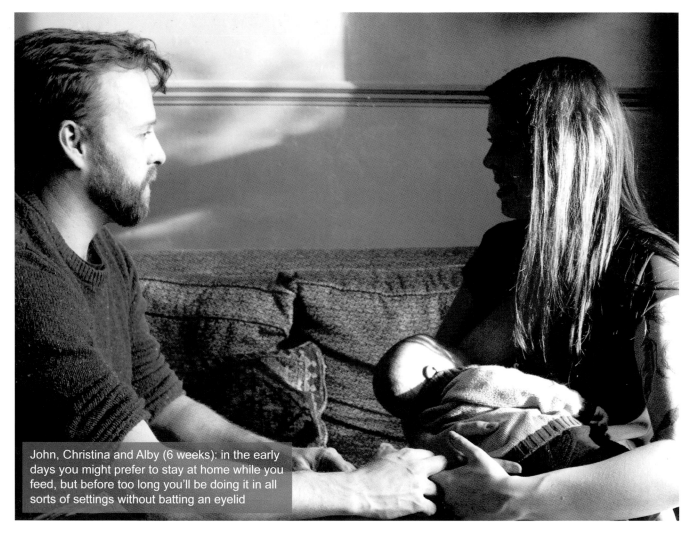

John, Christina and Alby (6 weeks): in the early days you might prefer to stay at home while you feed, but before too long you'll be doing it in all sorts of settings without batting an eyelid

The truth about breastfeeding

A lot of new breastfeeding mums say: "I wish someone had told me how hard it can be" and "I wasn't prepared for how difficult it is!" Breastfeeding is beautifully natural, fulfilling and rewarding, but it can also be painful during the early days before your nipples toughen up, and especially if your little one is teething. It can be physically tiring, and take up a lot of time. Staying hydrated and eating a varied diet with plenty of fresh fruit and veg can help with the exhaustion. Include iron-rich snacks such as dried apricots, seeds, prunes, dates and raisins.

During the early weeks of breastfeeding, you might notice some cramping as your womb contracts back to its former size. The act of breastfeeding helps this along due to the release in oxytocin, the great bonding and feel-good hormone, but it can initially feel rather intense. Being prepared and breathing through it can help. The oxytocin released during breastfeeding also makes your post partum bleeding lighter. If you are bottle-feeding, remember that hugs are a great way to release oxytocin.

It pays to gently remind yourself that it will take a little time for your womb to go back, whether you are breastfeeding or not. Even a day or two after the birth, your womb will have reduced to the size it was when you were around 18 weeks pregnant. After one week, your womb will have shrunk further to the size it was at the end of the first trimester, and by six weeks postpartum it should be pretty much as it was prior to the birth.

In the days following the birth, people will be far too enchanted by your little one to notice and no one will expect you to be back in your jeans. Just be sure that you don't judge yourself, as the last thing you need with a new baby is to be worrying about how you look. Take the time to enjoy the focus on your baby rather than your appearance.

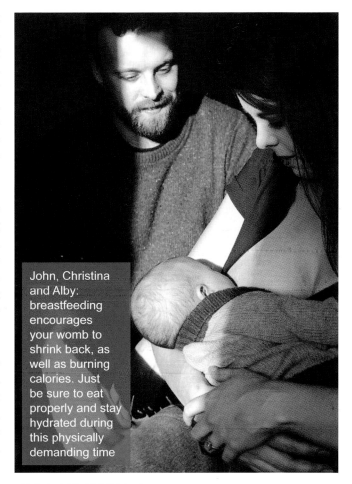

John, Christina and Alby: breastfeeding encourages your womb to shrink back, as well as burning calories. Just be sure to eat properly and stay hydrated during this physically demanding time

Holly: "I first fed Jasmine soon after the birth, when we were alone in the hospital bed. There was no audience and no pressure. Much later a midwife came round and said she was going to show me how to feed my baby. She looked sceptical when I explained that I had already done so and made me show her. I think trusting your natural instincts and letting your baby show you the way counts for a great deal."

Tongue-tie

Tongue-tie (ankyloglossia) is the name given to the birth defect in which a small tight piece of skin has formed between the floor of the mouth and the tongue. Even if you have a lot of experience with children, you may not be able to detect a tongue-tie just by looking at the tongue.

A baby with tongue-tie can struggle to latch on or can slip off the nipple when trying to feed. This is because babies with tongue-tie are unable to open their mouths wide enough to latch on to both the nipple and the breast tissue. If your nipples are sore and you have bleeding or ulcers, then a simple procedure can be carried out that will divide the tongue-tie and allow you to feed your baby.

Bottle-fed babies with tongue-tie are often hard to spot, but restricted tongue movement may mean that your baby is unable to seal the teat properly and may leak milk out of the corner of their mouth or take in a lot of air when they feed. They will struggle to feed, take a long time about it and may even fall asleep regularly at the bottle through exhaustion. They may also be colicky and suffer from trapped wind.[5]

Tongue-tie that does not affect feeding is often not treated or may even go undetected. It is only when a child starts to speak that a speech therapist may pick up on the reason behind their difficulties.

Back to work

If you are still breastfeeding when you go back to work, you will need to find somewhere comfortable to express milk, or your milk supply may stop. You shouldn't have to lock yourself away in the toilets to express, which may not be hygenic.

The law in the UK requires an employer to provide somewhere for a breastfeeding employee to rest, but not to grant paid breaks from a job in order to breastfeed or to express milk.[6] It is good practice to discuss your requirements with your employer before you return to work if possible. Ask your manager if there is a room you can use to express milk that is quiet and private. In New Zealand, employers are required to provide appropriate facilities and unpaid breaks for employees who want to breastfeed or express milk.[7] In Australia, there is legislation in place in most states to protect employees from being discriminated against on the grounds of family responsibility. The Australian Breastfeeding Association offer advice and can recommend discussing possible options with your employer.[8] For Canadian women the right to breastfeed whenever and wherever they need to is protected by the Canadian Charter of Rights. Although there is no specific legislation in place regarding breastfeeding at work, organizations such as Infant Feeding Action Coalition Canada (INFACT) are available to offer support and guidance.[9] In the USA the Affordable Care Act of 2010 requires employers to provide reasonable break time and facilities (other than a bathroom) for a woman to express breast milk until her child is one year old.[10]

Final thoughts

It is completely ok to admit if you need help, and if you are too tired to feed or think it is too painful or difficult then you might just need a little guidance. Whether you are feeding by bottle or breast, allow yourself this time to marvel at your baby and just relax. Although it may not feel marvellous during the wee hours when the rest of the family are happily sleeping, during the daytime a breastfeeding session can be really special time together for you and your wonderful new baby.

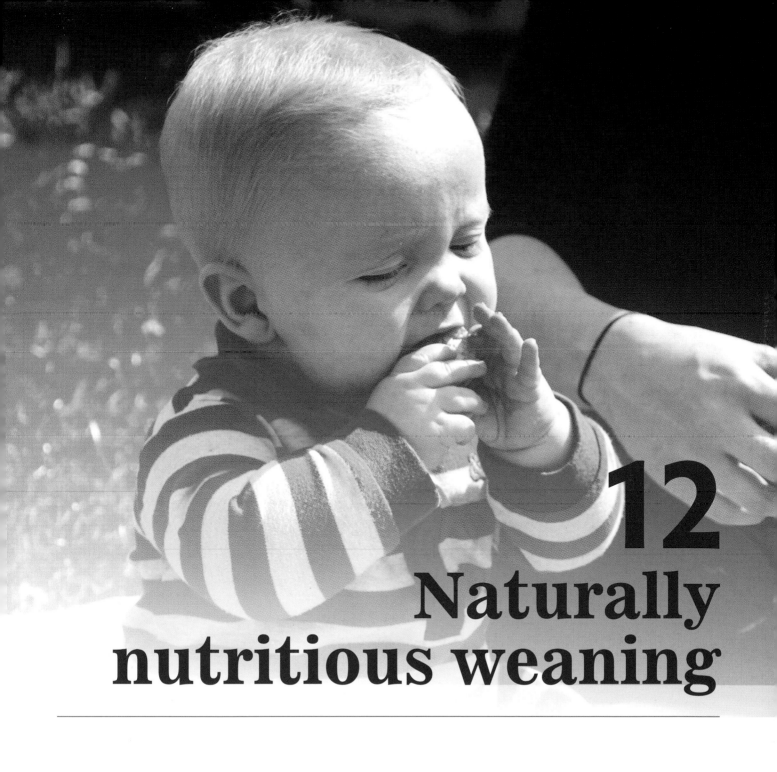

12 Naturally nutritious weaning

12
Naturally nutritious weaning

For the first six months, breast milk or infant formula milk provides all the nutrients that your baby needs.[1] And of course, those lovely calm feeding times, when your baby nestles close to you, are equally important in terms of their emotional development. Therefore, it's natural to feel slightly apprehensive when you begin weaning your baby from full breast-feeding or bottle-feeding towards a diet that includes solid foods. After all, by the time your baby shows signs of readiness for weaning, they have probably already settled into cosy feeding routines that are easy, relaxed and enjoyable for both of you. You might wonder how your baby will react to foods that have strange new flavours and unfamiliar lumpy textures. How can you ensure they receive a healthy, balanced diet? What types of foods should you offer first? Which foods should you avoid?

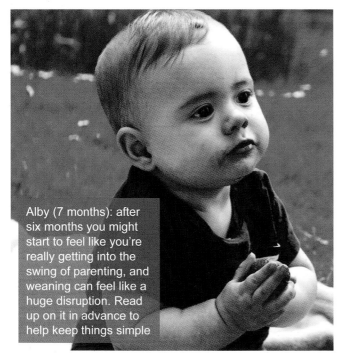

Alby (7 months): after six months you might start to feel like you're really getting into the swing of parenting, and weaning can feel like a huge disruption. Read up on it in advance to help keep things simple

This chapter aims to help you wean your baby on to a nutritious and well-balanced diet while keeping things relaxed – and fun.

Signs of readiness to wean

Research shows that babies can get all the nutrients they need from breast milk or infant formula until they are around 6 months old. Waiting till then gives their digestive system time to develop fully so that it can cope with solid food.[2] Earlier weaning could upset your baby's immature digestive system (and that means even more dirty laundry and nappy changes – no thanks!). You may find that some parents try to start their babies on baby rice as early as 4 or 5 months, but just ignore the baby Olympics where some parents seem eager to prove that their child is ahead of the pack. It's important to wait as the digestion system usually isn't mature enough prior to 6 months to handle a radical change.

So bide your time until your baby can hold their head steady and sit up comfortably, and look for signs of hand–eye coordination, where they can pick up small pieces of soft food and move them to their mouth. Also by the age of 6 months, your baby will be more adept at swallowing the foods you offer, rather than dribbling everything back out again!

Some signs that can be mistaken for a baby being ready for solid foods are:

- Chewing fists
- Waking in the night when they have previously slept through
- Wanting extra milk feeds.

These are normal behaviours and not necessarily signs of hunger. Starting solid foods won't make a baby any more likely to sleep through the night.[3]

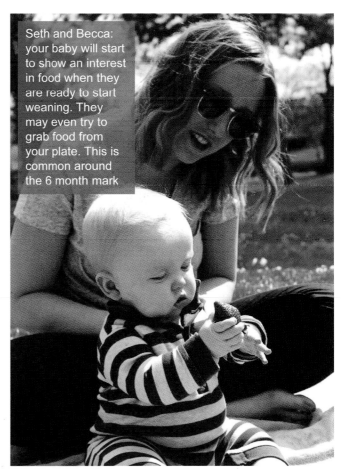

Seth (6 months): every new stage of your baby's development can feel a little scary, so focus instead on the miracle of their changing needs and embrace the growth

Seth and Becca: your baby will start to show an interest in food when they are ready to start weaning. They may even try to grab food from your plate. This is common around the 6 month mark

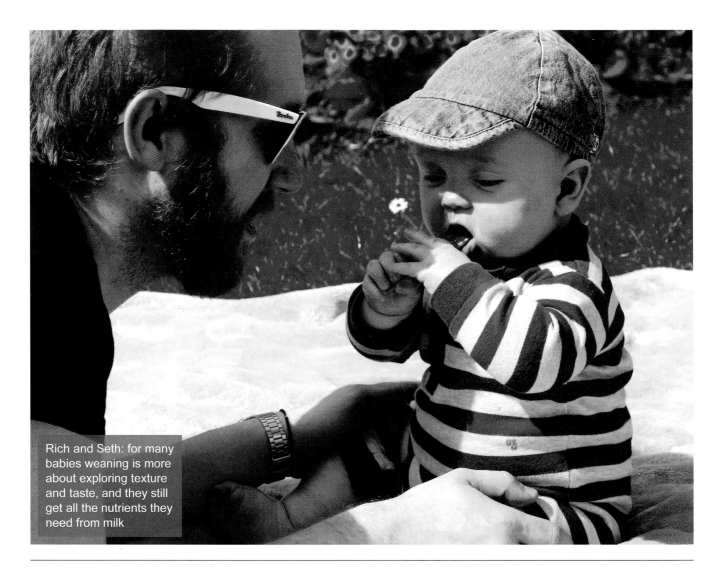

Rich and Seth: for many babies weaning is more about exploring texture and taste, and they still get all the nutrients they need from milk

Holly: "I made little frozen batons of banana so she could chomp down on them to soothe her gums while teething. As well as offering relief, the batons got munched up and swallowed. That was a very clear sign that she was ready to start weaning."

Baby's nutritional needs

The process of weaning your baby should be a slow transition. You can gradually reduce your baby's intake of breast milk or formula as they begin to accept wholesome meals.

At first, the focus of weaning your baby is to encourage them to explore different tastes and textures and master the mechanics of eating by learning how to chew and swallow foods with ease. Early days of weaning might sometimes resemble a sip-and-spit-out wine-tasting event. It might seem that your baby doesn't like a particular food if they push it back out with their tongue. However, it's more likely that they have yet logged a new food taste into their expanding memory of tastes. After all, prior to weaning your baby will have tasted only milk, and strange foods, especially if they taste bitter or sour, might provoke an instinctive adverse reaction. In terms of survival of the species, it could be said that an instinctive rejection deters babies from swallowing toxic substances such as poisonous berries or spoiled milk.

Try not to give too much credence to any of your baby's seeming likes and dislikes. Babies who are continually offered sweet-tasting foods, because that's what they seem to prefer, are likely to develop a taste for sweetness and may increasingly reject healthier alternatives. We can help babies to accept a range of tastes by offering any foods they initially reject in smaller quantities, or by combining them with naturally sweet foods. We should never coat food with extra sugar or salt, and there's no need to hide vegetables in meals as if they were criminal fugitives!

A relaxed manner and gentle persistence at your baby's meal times helps encourage a taste for well-balanced meals.

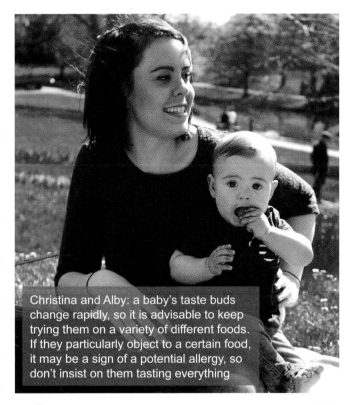

Christina and Alby: a baby's taste buds change rapidly, so it is advisable to keep trying them on a variety of different foods. If they particularly object to a certain food, it may be a sign of a potential allergy, so don't insist on them tasting everything

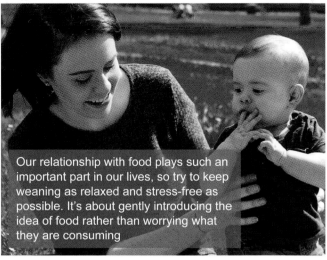

Our relationship with food plays such an important part in our lives, so try to keep weaning as relaxed and stress-free as possible. It's about gently introducing the idea of food rather than worrying what they are consuming

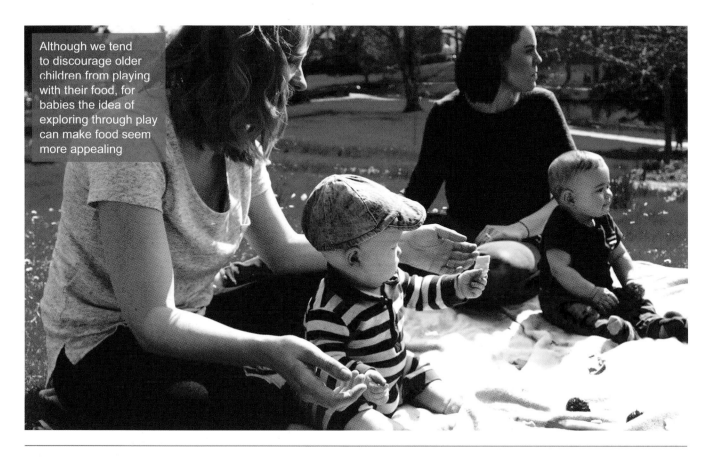

Although we tend to discourage older children from playing with their food, for babies the idea of exploring through play can make food seem more appealing

Holly: "I cooked extra veg while preparing dinner, puréed some up immediately and served it to her while we had our dinner. This got her into the idea of dinner times. I would then freeze the rest. Taste buds regenerate every 10-14 days, so if your baby isn't keen on a flavour now it is worth trying again. I think babies are more likely to try food if they are offered a few different varieties to play with. Lay them out on the tray of the high chair and let them explore for themselves without intervening with a spoon. This is baby-led weaning."

Babies are curious little souls who learn about the world through stimulation of their senses, including their sense of taste. This chapter aims to help you offer nutritious meals that will excite your baby's taste buds and expand their taste habits.

Above all, there's no need to stress if your baby seems pernickety and doesn't take much in at meal times. Breast milk or formula feeds provide sufficient amounts of protein, carbohydrates, fats, vitamins and minerals to meet your baby's needs at least until the age of 12 months, by which time they will be enjoying well-balanced meals and can be offered full-fat cow's milk instead. If you continue to breastfeed throughout the weaning period, you will ensure your baby receives sufficient calories and nutrients from your own well-balanced food choices. Breast milk also contains antibodies and enzymes that help boost your baby's immune system and protect them from illness and allergies.

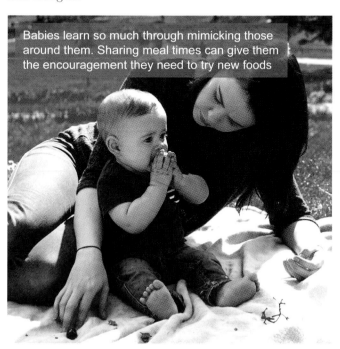

Babies learn so much through mimicking those around them. Sharing meal times can give them the encouragement they need to try new foods

Food essentials

Many parents worry that their children aren't eating a balanced diet as children can be rather fussy with their food. Introducing them to a variety of different foods now may help them to experiment later on.

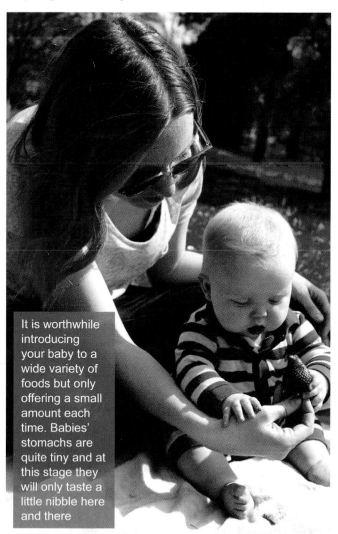

It is worthwhile introducing your baby to a wide variety of foods but only offering a small amount each time. Babies' stomachs are quite tiny and at this stage they will only taste a little nibble here and there

Protein

Proteins are essential to your baby's healthy growth and development. Protein comprises long chains of substances called amino acids, of which approximately twenty have so far been identified (with unattractive names such as lysine, arginine and tryptophan). Ten of these amino acids are not produced by the body and must be obtained from the foods we eat. Foods such as meat, fish and poultry are sources of complete protein because they contain all the essential amino acids we need.[4]

A note about fat and fibre

Unlike many adults, who may reap health benefits from a low-fat, high-fibre diet, babies have tiny tummies and can only take in small amounts of food at each meal time. Bulky foods, such as wheat bran and brown rice, may not provide sufficient calories and nutrients to meet your baby's needs for energy and growth. Offer full-fat dairy foods, such as whole milk and full-fat yogurts, to ensure sufficient fat and fat-soluble vitamins such as vitamin A and vitamin D. (Avoid high-fat foods that have little nutritive value, such as chips and cakes.)

Allergies

If you have a family history of food allergies, or your baby has been diagnosed with eczema or asthma, you might worry that they will develop an allergic reaction to certain foods. The likeliest allergens include peanuts, eggs, seeds, milk, soya, wheat and other foods that contain gluten, such as oats, rye and barley.[5]

It's a good idea to offer a small amount of a new food to your baby and then leave a gap of about three days to check for any signs of allergic reaction before introducing a different food. Common symptoms of food allergy include hives, swelling of the skin, dry skin, itchiness, breathing difficulties, wheezing, coughing and nasal congestion. If your baby shows unusual symptoms after eating a newly introduced food, it's best to remove that food from their diet and consult your doctor.

Worrisome foods
Honey

Honey is cleverly produced by wonderful bees – but don't offer it to your beautiful baby until they are at least 12 months old. Honey might harbour bacteria that could infect your baby's intestines and cause a serious illness known as infant botulism. (Honey is also high in sugar and is therefore best limited or avoided beyond the age of 12 months to protect your infant's teeth.)

Raw or undercooked eggs

Give your baby hard-boiled eggs to avoid the risk of food poisoning from nasties such as salmonella.

Salty foods

Excess salt is bad news for kidneys and is linked with high blood pressure, stomach cancer, osteoporosis and strokes. So factor in the salt content of any processed foods that you buy, such as baked beans and stock cubes.

Sugary foods

Tooth decay, risk of childhood obesity or developing heart disease and diabetes – enough said!

An exciting milestone has arrived – it's time for your baby's first foods

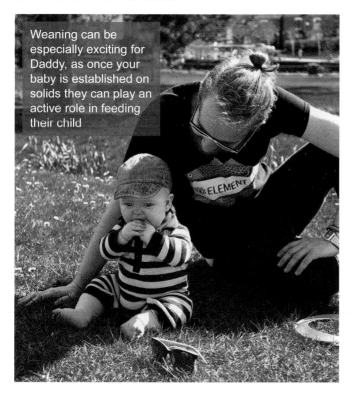

Weaning can be especially exciting for Daddy, as once your baby is established on solids they can play an active role in feeding their child

Step 1

- ### How do we start the weaning process?

Once your health visitor or health professional has advised you that your baby is ready for weaning, choose a specific area in your home to feed your baby. Babies prefer routine and will soon associate this chosen place with trying solid food (and hopefully the excitement that comes from experimenting with their culinary tastes).

Choose a quiet time when you are not rushed so you can give your baby your full attention. Give their usual milk feed first: you don't want your baby to be hungry when introducing food for the first time, but you don't want them to be full either.

Give yourself enough time to sit down with your baby and enjoy this whole process. If you are fitting in weaning between other commitments, you may begin to feel frustrated or anxious if your baby seems to reject all of your offerings. Let your baby explore the food you are offering and rather than just giving them purée on a spoon, allow them to play with it too. Baby-led weaning (letting the baby choose from a selection of different foods on their tray) may help take the pressure off. (For more information go to www.babyledweaning.com.)

The best time to wean your baby is when they are happy and alert. Make sure you have your bibs at hand and place a small amount of food into a bowl. First tastes should be mild and smooth in texture, which is why health

Sam: "All three of my kids tried to grab the spoon while I was trying to wean them. This led to a terrible mess and a frustrated Mummy and baby, until I gave them a spoon to play with."

professionals have always advised that a little plain baby rice mixed with your breast milk or formula (forming a runny blend) will be easy for babies to digest and accept as a new food source.

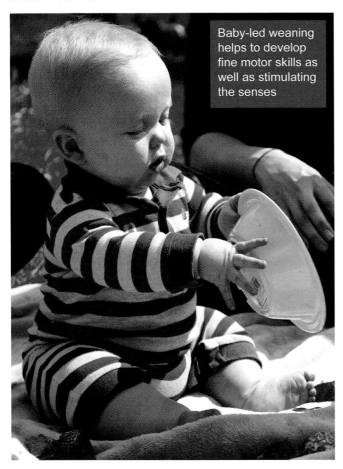

Baby-led weaning helps to develop fine motor skills as well as stimulating the senses

Once you have blended the rice and baby milk, offer a little to the child on the tip of a spoon. At 6 months a baby's tongue and mouth should be developed enough for dealing with food, but it may take some time for them to get the coordination to master this new skill. Don't be surprised if the food tends to come back out again in the early stages; your patience will be rewarded.

Step 2

Food to try feeding your child after baby rice should ideally be some sort of root vegetable, preferably steamed and then puréed. Cooked and puréed carrots can be easily digested by your baby's undeveloped digestive system. Babies should acquire the taste of vegetables first, so that they get used to their relative sourness. (Once you have established your baby eating their greens, you can move on to fruit purées.) Great first-try vegetable purées include: carrot, potato, swede, parsnip, pumpkin, butternut squash and sweet potato. These foods will nourish your baby while their naturally sweet flavours make them more appealing and easier to digest.

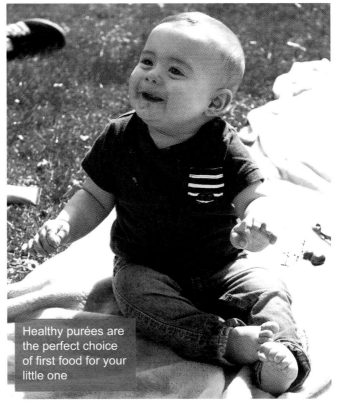

Healthy purées are the perfect choice of first food for your little one

It is important to give your baby time to adjust and get used to each new taste. You may wish to try mixing a little of your breast or formula milk into your baby's purées to make the transition stage more familiar.

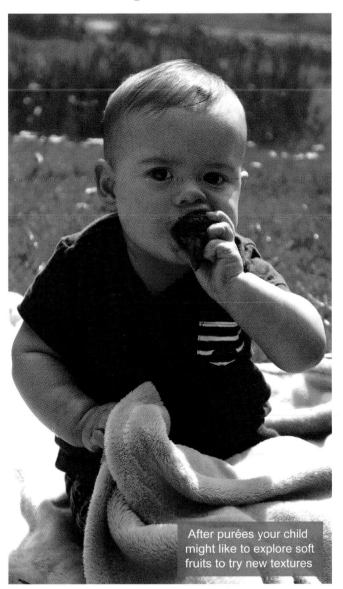

After purées your child might like to explore soft fruits to try new textures

Don't give up if your baby doesn't like something one day. Persist or try blending two ingredients together. It is important to take things slow and follow your baby's lead. Try as many different tastes as possible, and in time – however long this may take – your baby will have a nourishing, healthy and varied diet. Don't be too quick to compare notes: there will always be a baby in your social circle who readily eats everything put in front of them without a fuss. Babies develop their tastes in their own time.

The recipes that follow are just a guide, and, as with any cooking, there aren't any hard and fast rules; you can change and adapt the recipes to suit your child's taste and your convenience.

Handy recipes for weaning

Baby rice

Baby rice is the most recommended of first baby foods, but when shop-bought there are often added ingredients. Your baby doesn't need all those extras – they are getting all the additional benefits from milk. So why not make your very own version? It's great knowing exactly what you are feeding your little one, plus it's so easy to make. Baby rice can be frozen, so go ahead and make a big batch of it for future use.

Wash 2 tbsp of short-grain white rice (don't use brown rice at this stage as a baby's gut can't digest it) under running water until it is completely clean. Pop it into a small saucepan and top up with enough boiling water to cover. Stir once, then cover and simmer gently for half an hour or so. Once the rice is mushy, drain and purée with breast milk until it's a lovely creamy consistency.

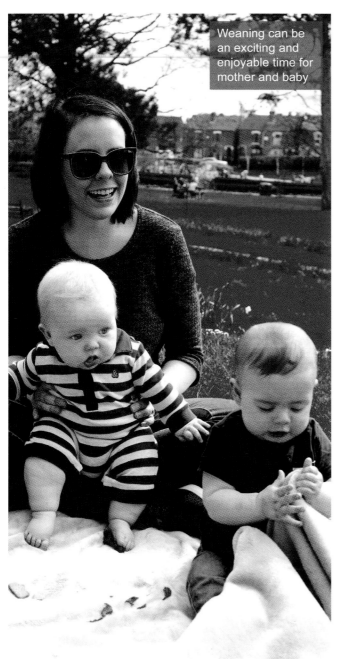

Weaning can be an exciting and enjoyable time for mother and baby

Basic vegetable purées

Root vegetables are sweet, full of nutrients and you can freeze what you don't use for later (perhaps in an ice-cube tray).

Carrots

Perhaps the most popular – for adults and babies – of all the root vegetables. Sweet and delicious and jam-packed full of antioxidants, dietary fibre and a multitude of vitamins (especially vitamin A, which is essential for enabling a healthy immune system, promoting growth and boosting vision, although it also contains much vitamin C, which is fantastic for maintaining teeth, gums and connective tissue). One carrot provides your baby with everything they need to stay healthy and thrive.

1 medium carrot (makes 4 portions)

Thoroughly wash the carrot and peel. Steam for 15 minutes. Purée until smooth and add breast milk (or formula) to create the perfect consistency.

Butternut squash

Butternut squash is easily digestible, high in vitamin A and mineral-rich, making it the perfect super-food for your baby.

½ butternut squash (makes 8-10 portions)

Peel the butternut squash, chop into cubes, and steam for 15 minutes or so. Purée the squash and add as much breast milk or formula as you require to give it a creamy texture.

Parsnips

Similar to carrots in their sweetness, these fabulous veggies are a good source of fibre, and vitamins C, E (a natural antioxidant) and K (excellent for blood clotting, and therefore healing wounds faster). Parsnips also contain folic acid, thiamin, pantothenic acid, copper, calcium, iron, potassium and manganese, all of which contribute to healthy bodies and minds.

1 parsnip (makes 6 portions)

Peel the parsnip and chop. Steam for around 15 minutes or so. Once cooked, purée to a smooth consistency, adding as much breast milk or formula as you require to get the perfect texture.

Sweet potatoes

Sweet potatoes are full of vitamins, minerals and antioxidants, and because they are a high-calorie vegetable they are especially good for weaning.

1 sweet potato (makes 6 portions)

Wash and scrub the skin and dry it thoroughly. Prick it all over with a fork. Pop it in the oven for about 45 minutes at 200°C (400°F / Gas Mark 6) until it's soft. Once cooked (and slightly cooled), split the skin and scoop out the inside. Mash it until smooth, adding breast milk or formula.

Pumpkins

Not just for Halloween, the pumpkin is an all-round brilliant vegetable since it is full of antioxidants, minerals (copper, calcium, potassium and phosphorus) and vitamins (vitamins A, B, B6, C and E).

1 small pumpkin (makes up to 10 portions)

Peel the pumpkin and chop. Steam on the hob for about 20 minutes (until tender). Purée the pumpkin until smooth, adding breast milk or formula.

Basic fruit purées

Once your baby's taste buds have mastered the taste of vegetables it's time to move on to sweeter foods.

Apples

Apples include a range of healthy vitamins and minerals including antioxidants and phytonutrients, and they boost the immune system.

1 small eating apple (makes 4 portions)

Wash the apple thoroughly, peel, core and chop. Pop the chunks into a steamer and steam until tender (for about

---

Holly: "Ice-cube trays are ideal for freezing tiny portions of freshly puréed veg. You can store them in freezer bags and label them. I used to combine a couple of cubes of different vegetables to keep things varied and interesting."

5 minutes or so). Purée until smooth and add breast milk or formula if you choose (this isn't necessary, but you might want to for flavour and consistency).

• •

Bananas

Bananas are packed full of vitamin B6 and vitamin C, as well as copper, potassium and manganese (which is fabulous for strengthening bones). They not only taste incredible, but the texture is already lovely and soft, so they are easy to prepare and digest.

¼ small banana (makes 1 portion)

Mash the banana with a fork, getting rid of all the lumps. Add enough milk (both breast milk and formula work equally well) to give it a smooth texture.

• •

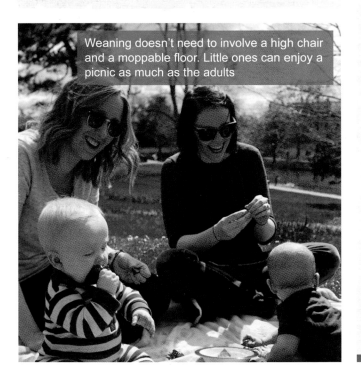

Weaning doesn't need to involve a high chair and a moppable floor. Little ones can enjoy a picnic as much as the adults

Pears

Pears tend to get a little forgotten about, maybe because they need to be ripe. That's a shame, as not only do they taste great, but also they are super-good for you. Pears have loads of minerals (copper, iron, potassium, manganese and magnesium), as well as folates (where folic acid comes from) and riboflavin (essential for red-blood cell production).

1 small ripe pear (makes 4 portions)

Wash the pear, peel and core it. Put it in a saucepan with a little bit of water, and bring to the boil. Once boiling, turn down the heat and simmer (covered) for around 7 minutes. Once soft, purée and add breast milk or formula.

• •

Mangoes

Mangoes, possibly the most summery of fruits, are vitamin-filled, juicy and delicious.

1 small mango (makes 6 portions)

Wash and peel to get as much of the flesh as possible. Cut it away from the centre stone and purée.

• •

Avocados

Avocados are rich in dietary fibre, minerals, nutrients and vitamins. They pretty much have everything your weaning baby could possibly want.

½ medium ripe avocado (makes 3 portions)

Simply mash the flesh of the avocado until it's as smooth as it will go, and then add breast milk or formula to get it to the right consistency.

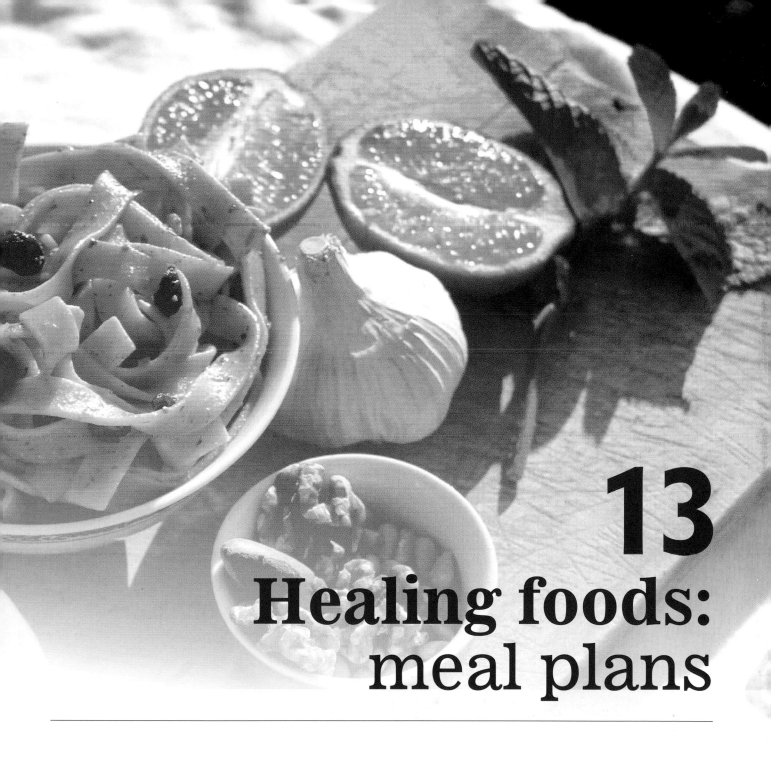

13
Healing foods: meal plans

13
Healing foods: meal plans

The best time to start preparing for a holistic pregnancy (and childbirth) is before you conceive. Being well yourself impacts on your baby's health, and being in good health gives you a much better chance of conceiving in the first place. Good news all round!

Pregnancy can make women feel unwell for some or all of the 40 weeks, and even common ailments can feel much worse due to a debilitated immune system, so understanding how to get the right balance of nutrients in your food is all-important.

Our bodies are amazing. We can fight fatigue, boost our immune systems, and generally fix ourselves right up (including when pregnant) with the foods that we eat. The following recipes are suitable at any stage, including during pregnancy.

Note for Australian readers:

An Australian tablespoon is 20ml (⅔fl oz), as opposed to the more standard 15ml (½fl oz). Readers using Australian measures should therefore use 3 x 5ml teaspoons to obtain a tablespoon in the following recipes.

Foods to fight fatigue

Breakfast: porridge oats with blueberries and cinnamon

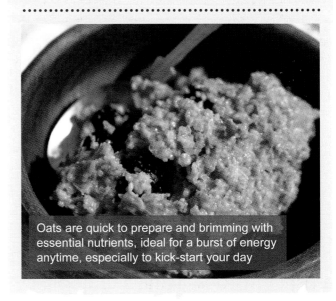

Oats are quick to prepare and brimming with essential nutrients, ideal for a burst of energy anytime, especially to kick-start your day

The ingredients in this breakfast are just magical. Porridge oats give you a slow release of energy and fibre, and their nutrients help to support a healthy nervous system. They also include a natural sedative, the alkaloid gramine, which will improve your mood and keep you calm. Add blueberries (an acknowledged super-food) to these oats to help energize you for your day ahead.

Serves 1

50g (1¾oz) porridge oats

270ml (9fl oz) milk

1 tsp (ground) cinnamon

75g (just over 2½oz) blueberries

Pour the oats into a saucepan and add the milk. Bring to the boil and allow to simmer for 4-5 minutes. Stir in the cinnamon and blueberries and serve warm.

Lunch: sweet potato and carrot soup

Sweet potatoes are excellent for combating fatigue since they contain loads of slow-digesting carbohydrates (much more than regular potatoes). As a bonus, they help strengthen the immune system since they are rich in beta carotene and vitamin C. These nutrients (also found in carrots) ramp up your energy levels to give you a good boost.

Serves 4

1 tbsp coconut oil / rapeseed oil

2 shallots (sliced)

4 tbsp water

4 large carrots (chopped)

2 garlic cloves (crushed)

1 sweet potato (cubed)

500ml (18fl oz) vegetable stock

Heat the coconut oil in a saucepan over a medium heat and add the shallots. Cook them for 2-3 minutes until soft. Next, add the water, carrots, garlic and sweet potato and sweat them for 4-5 minutes. If the sweet potato starts to discolour, remove from the heat. Once cooked, add the stock and simmer for 15 minutes.

Allow to cool slightly and then blend to a smooth consistency using a food processor or blender. You can serve the soup straight away, or keep it in the fridge for later.

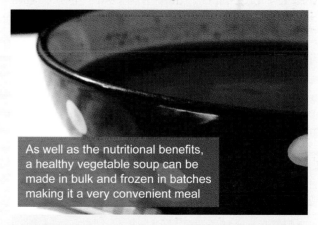

As well as the nutritional benefits, a healthy vegetable soup can be made in bulk and frozen in batches making it a very convenient meal

Dinner: mushroom risotto

Mushrooms are a natural mood enhancer. They increase the body's oxygen-carrying capacity and fight adrenal fatigue, which is why they perk us up. They also contain a

Sam: "This is a perfect recipe to batch cook, making it quick and easy to get an energy boost in the afternoon."

lot of vitamin B, which enables our bodies to really use all the energy they can from the food we consume. Healthy skin, digestion and nerves all stem from good levels of vitamin B. Mushrooms contain a lot of B vitamins such as riboflavin, niacin and pantothenic acid, all of which promote energy levels.

Serves 4

500ml (18fl oz) chicken stock

1 tbsp olive oil

1 large onion (chopped)

200g (7oz) mushrooms (sliced)

2 garlic cloves (minced)

240g (8½oz) risotto rice

Salt and pepper

80g (2¾oz) parmesan (grated)

15g (½oz) parsley (chopped)

Make the chicken stock as per the pack instructions, and leave to one side. (For a low-salt alternative you can make your own by simmering a deep pan of water into which you have added a chicken carcass, garlic, seasoning and herbs for 3-4 hours. You'll need to skim the surface regularly to remove bitter fat. There are plenty of recipes for homemade stock available online.) In a medium saucepan or wok heat the oil and add the onion, mushrooms and garlic. Cook until softened (about 2-3 minutes). Pour in the risotto rice and then gradually add the stock a little at a time. Stir constantly until the rice is tender (20-25 minutes). Remove from the heat, season, stir in the parmesan and parsley, and serve, garnished with parsley.

Other foods that help to fight fatigue are fish, beans, wholegrain, and fruit and veg with high vitamin C content (such as citrus fruits, peppers and broccoli).

Increased immunity

Breakfast: berry burst smoothie

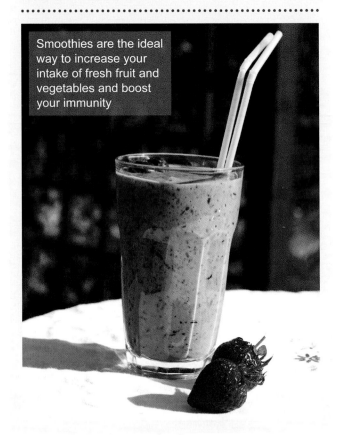

Smoothies are the ideal way to increase your intake of fresh fruit and vegetables and boost your immunity

Holly: "Risotto can be a strong weaning choice for an older baby; just replace the salty stock with coconut milk for more flavour."

This smoothie is one of the very best when it comes to giving your immune system a big boost. The fruits combat the toxic free radicals in your body, and also included are tons of vitamin C and E, polyphenols, selenium and zinc. Everything in this smoothie is high in antioxidants.

Serves 2

237ml (8½fl oz) coconut water

3 tbsp plain yoghurt

70g (2½oz) strawberries

70g (2½oz) blueberries

70g (2½oz) raspberries

1 tsbp chia seeds

Pop everything into a blender and whizz for around 30-45 seconds until smooth. Drink!

Lunch: chicken soup

Chicken soup is famous all over the world for its healing properties. It keeps the body hydrated, the vegetables boost your immune system, and the chicken has iron and protein.

Serves 4-6

1 medium whole chicken (cooked, skinned and shredded)

1 tbsp coconut oil

1 brown onion

1 leek

4 sticks of celery (chopped)

6 carrots (peeled and chopped)

1.2 litres (40fl oz) chicken stock

Salt and pepper

1 tbsp parsley (chopped)

While the chicken is cooking nicely, melt the coconut oil in a large saucepan over a medium heat. Throw in the onion, leek, celery and carrots and fry until they start to soften.

Pour in the chicken stock and bring the whole mixture to the boil, stirring all the time. Season, then reduce the heat and simmer for 10 minutes (or until the vegetables are tender).

Shred the cooked chicken (or do this earlier) and add to the soup. Keep cooking to heat it all through then serve with parsley as a garnish.

Dinner: Brazil nut pesto pasta

This lovely quick pasta dish has plenty to keep you healthy. Brazil nuts are a good source of the mineral selenium, which aids the immune system. You only need three or four Brazil nuts a day to get all the selenium you need. Walnuts are perfect for replacing fish in your diet as they are a great source of omega-3s.[1]

Serves 2-4

2 tbsp pinenuts

6 Brazil nuts

2 tbsp walnuts

50g (1¾oz) fresh basil leaves

1 tbsp mint leaves

3 tbsp parmesan (grated)

125ml (4½fl oz) olive oil

A dash of lime

3 garlic cloves

400g (14oz) tagliatelle pasta

140g (5oz) sultanas

Place the pinenuts in a frying pan and cook on low heat for 2-3 minutes. Allow to cool and then pop them in a food processor along with the Brazil nuts, walnuts, basil, mint, parmesan, olive oil, lime and garlic. Whizz it all up until smooth.

Cook the pasta according to the pack instructions and drain well. Return the pasta to the pan, stir in the homemade pesto and sultanas, season, and serve with a sprinkling of parmesan.

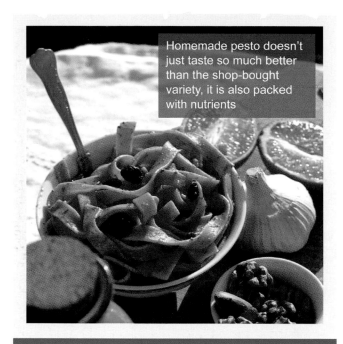
Homemade pesto doesn't just taste so much better than the shop-bought variety, it is also packed with nutrients

Stress and anxiety

Stress can be hard to avoid. If life feels a bit much, making time for self-care and adopting a stress-busting diet is the best way forward.

Breakfast: granola

Granola is made from oats and seeds and will kick-start your day like nothing else. The ingredients are renowned for supporting the nervous system during stressful situations; they actually affect the neurotransmitters in the body (including the hormone serotonin, which is why they leave you feeling so good). You'll also be less inclined to snack before lunch.

Serves 4-6

170g (6oz) rolled oats (or porridge oats)
55g (2oz) almonds (chopped)
55g (2oz) coconut (shredded)
55g (2oz) walnuts (chopped)
55g (2oz) flaxseeds
55g (2oz) pumpkin seeds
55g (2oz) sunflower seeds
2 tbsp coconut oil
3 tbsp honey
1 tsp cinnamon (ground)
2 tsp vanilla extract
55g (2oz) dried raisins
55g (2oz) dried cranberries

Preheat the oven to 180°C (350°F / Gas Mark 4). While it's heating up, combine the oats, nuts and seeds in a large bowl.

In a saucepan, combine the coconut oil, honey, cinnamon and vanilla. Heat the mixture gently until the honey is just soft and everything is mixed well together. Remove from the heat, pour over the oaty mixture, and combine well.

Line a baking tray with baking paper and spread the granola over it. Bake for 20-30 minutes, checking every 10 minutes and moving around on the tray if necessary (to ensure it all browns evenly). When the granola is golden-brown, take out of the oven and allow to cool. Add the raisins and cranberries. Serve with almond milk if possible and, if not all eaten at once, store in an airtight container.

Lunch: mushroom and tofu stirfry

This is one fully loaded lunch! Packed full of stress-busting food such as shiitake mushrooms (which are known for containing potent phytonutrients, allowing the body to become more resistant to stress and fatigue), it also includes foods that are full of vitamin B such as mangetout and mung bean sprouts.

Serves 4

400g (14oz) plain tofu (cubed)

2 tbsp coconut oil

5g (¼oz) fresh rice noodles

150g (5¼oz) shiitake mushrooms (sliced)

100g (3½oz) mung bean sprouts

1 red chilli (finely chopped)

100g (3½oz) mangetout (trimmed)

1 red pepper (sliced)

4 spring onions (chopped)

2 tbsp raw Coconut Aminos (soya-free sauce)

Fresh coriander (chopped)

Cut the tofu into chunks (about 3cm/1⅛" thick). Heat 1 tbsp of coconut oil in a wok and fry the tofu until it is golden-brown all over. This can be done in two batches if required. Transfer from the heat into a warm dish.

Meanwhile, cook the noodles as per the packet instructions.

Next, heat 1 tbsp of coconut oil in the wok, add the shiitake mushrooms and fry for 2-3 minutes. Set aside with the tofu and start cooking the mung bean sprouts, chilli, mangetout, red pepper and spring onions. It only takes a couple of minutes, then pour in the Coconut Aminos sauce. Mix the noodles through, separating them with a fork, add the mushrooms and tofu and stir briefly. Serve on a warm plate or bowl garnished with coriander.

● ●

Dinner: Fish pie with saffron mash

Fish is an excellent source of vitamin B, and vitamin B relieves the symptoms of stress. Added to this, fish is also rich in magnesium, which is known as the anti-stress mineral. Both chilli and saffron have anti-depressant properties.

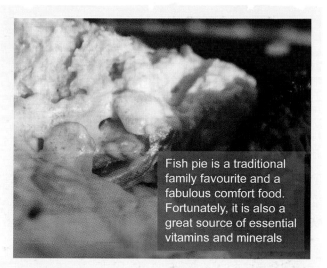

Fish pie is a traditional family favourite and a fabulous comfort food. Fortunately, it is also a great source of essential vitamins and minerals

Serves 4-6

25g (just over ¾oz) butter

25g (just over ¾oz) flour

1 leek (finely chopped)

400ml (14fl oz) milk

60g (2¼oz) cheese (grated)

1 pack of fish pie mix
(cod, salmon, smoked haddock etc. The weight should be around 400g/14oz)

1 tbsp Dijon mustard

1 tbsp thyme

600g (1lb 5oz) potatoes (peeled and halved)

100ml (3½fl oz) double cream

A dozen saffron threads (ground)

20g (¾oz) parsley (chopped)

Preheat the oven to 180°C (350°F / Gas Mark 4).

Place the butter, flour and leek into a pan and heat until the butter has melted. Stir as it cooks (about 1-2 minutes). Slowly whisk in the milk a little at a time (a balloon whisk is ideal). Bring the mixture to the boil and stir to remove lumps. Cook for another 3-4 minutes to allow it to thicken.

Remove from the heat and stir in the cheese, fish, mustard and thyme. Spoon everything into an oven-proof dish.

Cook the potatoes in boiling water until tender, then drain and mash. Set aside as you heat the cream and saffron in a saucepan. Once warmed, beat this into the mash as well. Smooth the mash over the top of the fish mixture, forking the surface once done. Bake for around 35 minutes until the potato is nice and golden. Garnish with parsley, and serve.

Other foods that combat stress are turkey, salmon, Greek yoghurt, and anything high in vitamin B such as eggs, soya beans, and leafy green veg.

Constipation

In pregnancy hormones can make us prone to constipation. Adding roughage to your diet will make all the difference. Here are some tasty recipes that will make eating more fibre seem a little bit more appealing..

Breakfast: berry crunch

Everything in this delicious and lovely-looking breakfast is good for constipation. Seeds are a gentle laxative and oats have plenty of fibre for roughage. The berries are full of super antioxidants and this, along with a good dollop of natural plain yoghurt, makes berry crunch the breakfast of healthy champions.

Serves 2

85g (3oz) wholegrain wheat flakes
35g (1¼oz) pumpkin seeds
35g (1¼oz) sunflower seeds
35g (1¼oz) linseeds (ground)
70g (2½oz) dried prunes (chopped)

100g (3½oz) mixed berries
1 tbsp plain yoghurt

Preheat the oven to 180°C (350°F / Gas Mark 4). Place the wheat flakes on a baking tray and bake for about 15 minutes. Turn occasionally to stop them from burning. Pour them into a large bowl and mix together with the pumpkin seeds, sunflower seeds and linseeds. Now mix the prunes and berries into the mixture. Serve with plain yoghurt on the top.

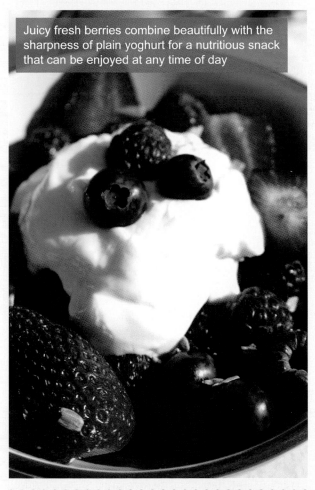

Juicy fresh berries combine beautifully with the sharpness of plain yoghurt for a nutritious snack that can be enjoyed at any time of day

Lunch: kale and sweet potato hotpot

Not only are sweet potatoes excellent at boosting your energy levels, they are also great at relieving constipation and are easy to digest. Bonus fact: they are a slow release of sugars, so they keep you active for longer, plus they boost serotonin levels. Serotonin is the brain chemical that makes you feel mellow and happy. You can't go wrong with a sweet potato! And did you know that kale is one of the most nutritious prenatal foods? This dark green leafy vegetable comes loaded with nutrients that are just right for your growing baby with an abundance of fibre, vitamins and calcium.

Serves 2
1 tbsp coconut oil
1 red onion (sliced)
2 garlic cloves (crushed)
1 tsp coriander seeds (crushed)
1 tsp chilli flakes
1 large sweet potato (peeled and cubed)
125g (4½oz) curly kale (finely chopped, without stalks)
Salt and pepper

Heat the coconut oil in a frying pan and add the onion. Fry gently. Once soft, add the garlic, coriander seeds and chilli flakes. Stir well. Next throw in the sweet potato and a little water. Cook everything for around 5 minutes, stirring constantly to stop the potato browning, pop in the kale and cook for another 5-8 minutes (until the potato is tender). Season and serve.

Dinner: bean curry

Pulses and beans are great for the digestive system, and may help relieve constipation and regulate bowel movements. Try serving this dish with brown rice, which increases energy levels and helps to sort out the immune system. Brown rice is a good source of magnesium, phosphorus, selenium, thiamine, niacin and vitamin B6, and an excellent source of manganese.[2]

Serves 4
1 tbsp coconut oil
1 red onion (finely chopped)
1 tsp cumin seeds
2 garlic cloves (crushed)
1 tin chopped tomatoes
1 tin chickpeas
1 tin kidney beans
2 tbsp medium curry powder
500g (1lb 1½oz) spinach
Fresh corriander (chopped)

Heat the coconut oil in a saucepan and fry the onion until soft. Add the cumin seeds, cook for another couple of minutes, and then add the garlic for the final minute of cooking. Pour on the tinned tomatoes and beans and stir well. Add the curry powder and keep stirring, and then pop in the spinach. Cook gently until the spinach has wilted. Serve with brown rice and sprinkle with fresh coriander.

Other foods that reduce constipation are figs, apricots, raisins, high-fibre cereals, broccoli, plums, pears and apples.

Anaemia

Anaemia is very common in pregnancy and with new mums; adding these iron-rich recipes into your weekly diet will help you to replenish your nutrients and feel more energetic.

Breakfast: spinach omelette

Iron-deficiency can lead to fatigue, tiredness and decreased immunity.[3] Spinach is packed with vitamins and minerals, and is one of the most iron-dense foods around. This means that the body can produce more energy to combat that debilitating feeling of tiredness.

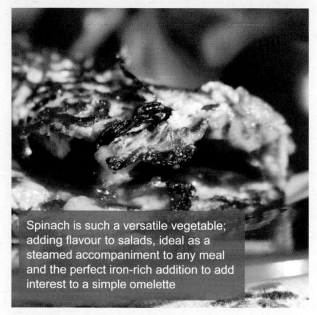

Spinach is such a versatile vegetable; adding flavour to salads, ideal as a steamed accompaniment to any meal and the perfect iron-rich addition to add interest to a simple omelette

Serves 1
55g (2oz) baby spinach
2 eggs
2 garlic cloves (crushed)
Salt and pepper
1 tbsp milk
1 tbsp olive oil
25g (over ¾oz) feta (or grated) cheese

Make sure the spinach is washed and then steam it until it has wilted. Set aside.

Break the eggs into a bowl and whisk – you want them frothy. Next, whisk in the garlic, salt and pepper and milk. Once combined, add the spinach and stir.

Heat a non-stick pan on a gentle heat and add in the olive oil to warm. Pour the egg mixture into the middle of the pan, tilting every now and then, and lifting the edges of the omelette as it starts to cook. This ensures that all of the egg bakes nicely. Cover the pan and cook for a further minute. Sprinkle cheese on the top, fold in half, and serve.

A great tip with this dish is to serve it with a glass of fresh orange juice as the vitamin C helps your body to absorb the iron.

• •

Lunch: chilli fish tacos

Halibut is a good source of iron if you're not keen on red meat. These tacos are ideal for a light snack at lunchtime.

Serves 2
2½ tsp chilli powder
2 tbsp lime juice
2 tbsp rapeseed oil
1 tsp cumin (ground)
4 garlic cloves (crushed)
Salt and pepper
2 pieces of halibut (around 115g/4oz each)

Holly: "Pregnancy, the birth itself and the weeks of blood loss (lochia) that follow can really take their toll, especially when combined with sleep deprivation. Remember to combine iron-rich foods with vitamin C to help with absorption. A supplement like spirulina might work well."

Holly: "Ginger and coconut are such a delicious and fragrant combination. Vegetarians might like to substitute the chicken for chickpea, tofu or tempeh, which are rich in protein and iron as well as being fantastic at absorbing flavour."

2 tbsp butter
1 tbsp flour
150ml (5¼fl oz) milk
50ml (1¾fl oz) sour cream
25g (just over ¾oz) chives
4 tacos

Preheat the oven to 180°C (350°F / Gas Mark 4). Combine the chilli powder, lime juice, oil, cumin, half the garlic, and salt and pepper in a bowl. Mix well, and then rub all over the fish. Wrap the fish in foil, place on a baking tray, and cook for 20-25 minutes.

While the fish is cooking, it's time to make the creamy chive sauce. Heat the butter in a pan and add the rest of garlic, frying it for a minute or so. Add the flour and mix well, then slowly add the milk, blending it with the flour until the mixture is smooth, creamy and thick. Add the sour cream and chives and set aside.

The fish will be done when the flesh flakes away easily with a fork. Transfer the fish to a plate, separate into chunks, and place in equal quantities in the tacos. Serve with a dollop of sauce on the top.

• •

Dinner: ginger coconut curry

This delicious curry will most certainly tantalize your taste buds. Chicken contains iron and protein, which when combined increases and restores your energy levels. This dish is ideal if you're suffering from anaemia.

Serves 4
1 tbsp coconut oil
1 medium onion (sliced)
1 tbsp cumin seeds
3 garlic cloves (crushed)
1 tbsp ginger (finely chopped)
1 red chilli
1 tsp garam masala
1 tsp turmeric
300ml (10½fl oz) coconut milk
3 chicken breasts (cubed)
½ chicken stock-cube
Salt and pepper
Fresh coriander (chopped)

Heat the coconut oil in a suacepan and fry the onion for 2-3 minutes, stirring as you go. Add the cumin seeds, garlic, ginger, chilli, garam masala and turmeric, and cook for another minute, stirring constantly. Next add the coconut milk and chicken and mix well. Finally crumble the stock-cube in and season. Bring to the boil then reduce the heat, cover, and simmer for about 20 minutes.

Serve with brown rice and a sprinkling of fresh coriander.

Other foods that help when you are anaemic are dark green leafy veg (such as watercress and curly kale), brown rice, nuts and seeds, white and red meat, and seafood. Beans and dried fruit are also rich in iron. Boost your iron intake by eating iron-rich foods together – a little meat can help you absorb more iron from beans and greens, or pair them with foods high in vitamin C.

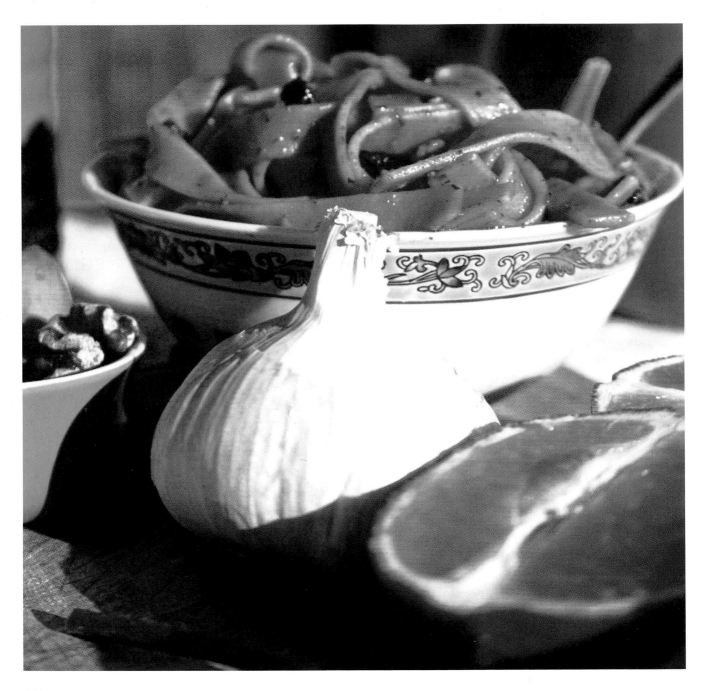

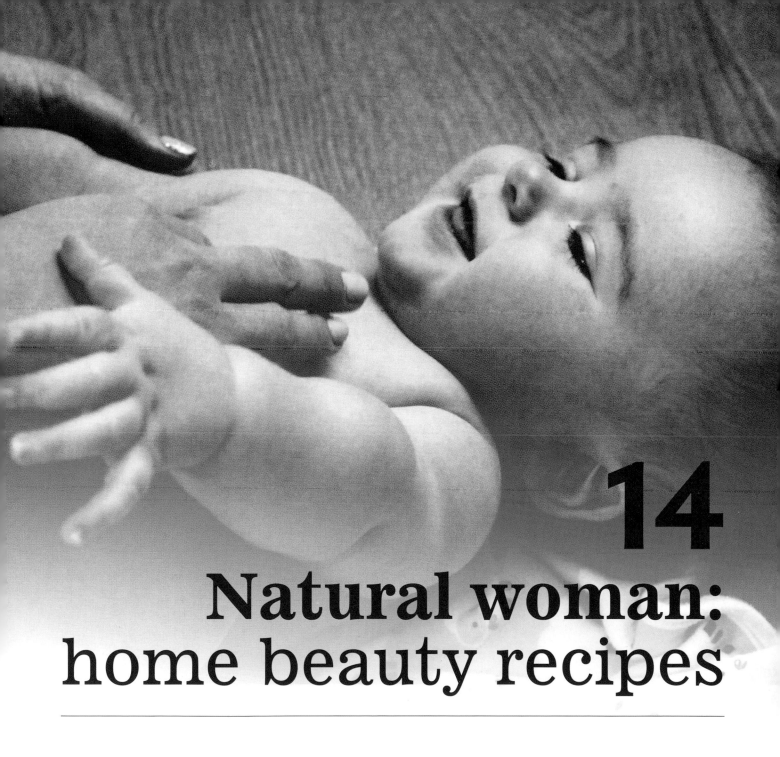

14

Natural woman:
home beauty recipes

14
Natural woman: home beauty recipes

Making your own beauty products can have many benefits. Hidden away in your cupboards and fridges may be vast treasures of natural beauty ingredients that could transform your skin and hair.

Here's some expert advice on how to include them in your beauty regime. These are completely chemical-free and won't tug on your purse strings.

Homemade hair care

Creating your own hair products means that you can limit the amount of chemicals that you come into contact with, and you can experiment with different fragrances. Natural ingredients are a lot of fun. Before too long you'll be concocting your own recipes for affordable and sustainable hair care products from home.

Homemade coconut shampoo

Coconut milk is used in Ayurvedic remedies. It truly is a gift from mother nature.

55ml (2fl oz) coconut milk
75ml (just over 2½fl oz) liquid Castile soap
1 tsp avocado oil
10 drops of chamomile essential oil

Combine all ingredients in a squeezy bottle or jar and shake well to mix. You can keep it in the fridge for up to a month. Give the mixture a good shake before every use.

Sam: "I love using this shampoo, it's wonderful for keeping hair in good condition. Women tend to lose hair after giving birth. This is natural, you are not going bald. When pregnant, the oestrogen in your body freezes hair in the growing phase, and the hair that would normally fall out stays put due to your pregnancy hormones. After birth your hormone levels drop along with your hair. This is only temporary, and it's simply hormonal."

Holly: "Sometimes when I am under a lot of pressure or have overdone the heat styling, my scalp goes quite flaky. I start with a 10-minute scalp massage with warm olive oil, followed by an exfoliating wash using a gentle shampoo with an added tablespoon of sugar and lukewarm water. Finally, I use a cup of apple cider vinegar with four drops of rosemary essential oil as a rinse."

Coconut hair mask

This treatment is so simple; all you have to do is apply the mixture to your hair. Applying the mixture nourishes the hair from root to tip. It will take less than 5 minutes to cover your hair.

1 ripe avocado
55ml (2fl oz) coconut milk
3 tsp coconut oil

Mash the avocado with a spoon until it's a smooth paste. Whisk in the coconut oil and milk, making sure they mix well into a lovely paste. Apply to your hair from roots to ends, massaging it into your scalp. Leave on for at least 30 minutes (overnight is ideal) and shampoo out.

Hair rinse

Apple cider vinegar's acidity can help improve porosity. The rinse works by sealing the hair cuticle, which helps the hair maintain more moisture and can result in a gorgeous shine.

6 tbsp (90ml / just over 3fl oz) apple cider vinegar
1 tbsp dried mint leaves
6 drops of lavender oil
475ml (16fl oz) water

Place vinegar, mint and oil in a pan, and pour the water over them. Simmer for around 10 minutes before letting the mixture cool completely. Strain. The rinse is now ready to use. Slowly pour through your hair after you've shampooed and conditioned. Leave hair for a few minutes before rinsing with cool or tepid water.

Fabulous facials

A visit to the spa is not always an option when there are little mouths to feed, and shop-bought products can be packed with chemicals or sport a hefty price tag.

Nourishing avocado face mask

This is the simplest but most beneficial face mask to make. Avocado is extremely nourishing for the skin, leaving it feeling vibrant and alive. Use organic avocado for the best results.

1 very ripe organic avocado

Peel the avocado and remove stone; mash in a small bowl until there are no lumps. Apply to a cleansed face for 10 minutes and rest. Wash off mask with warm water and moisturize.

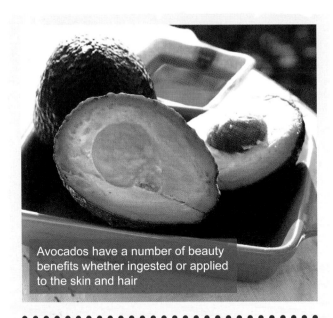

Avocados have a number of beauty benefits whether ingested or applied to the skin and hair

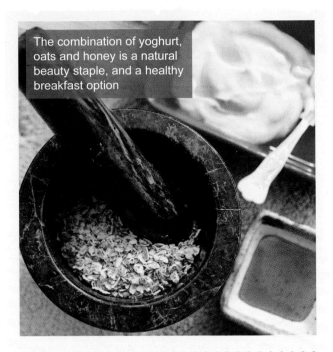

The combination of yoghurt, oats and honey is a natural beauty staple, and a healthy breakfast option

Oat and honey rejuvenating mask

We absolutely love this face mask. Honey is a humectant, so helps prevent loss of moisture in the skin. Oats contain antioxidants and anti-inflammatory compounds, which help soothe irritated skin.

1 tbsp manuka honey
1 tbsp Greek yogurt
1 tbsp oats (ground, ideally done in a coffee grinder)

Warm the honey slightly in a pan before adding the yogurt and ground oats. Whisk ingredients over a very low heat. Remove from the heat and allow to cool until the mask is warm enough to be comfortable to touch. Apply to your face for around 10 minutes before washing off and moisturizing.

Warning: always test the temperature of the mask before applying.

Banana and oat face mask

In the natural beauty world, bananas are known as nature's botox. Bananas protect the skin from free radicals, which are great for helping delay the ageing process. They are also packed full of vitamins and minerals essential for skin health. Combining bananas with oats helps soften the skin (when applied topically), keeping it in tip-top condition.

1 small banana
1 tbsp oats (ground)
1 tsp avocado oil

Blend the banana, oats and avocado oil in a blender. Apply to your face, and leave for around 10 minutes before washing off and moisturizing.

Honey and brown sugar facial scrub

We are in love with this softening facial scrub. Brown sugar is an excellent natural exfoliant. It doesn't tear the skin like salt can do and smells absolutely scrummy. Adding honey gives this scrub great cleansing properties. Honey is a very effective skin cleanser, drawing out impurities from the pores. Honey acts as a natural antibiotic and helps to pull dirt from skin pores by clearing blackheads. It hydrates and tightens skin pores for clear complexions.[1]

120ml (just over 4fl oz) honey
100g (3½oz) brown sugar
1 tbsp avocado oil

Mix together and apply the mixture to the face and massage in circular movements. This ensures you're removing dead skin from your face. Massage for around 5 minutes before rinsing well.

Anti-ageing facial oil (dry skin)

Avocado oil steals the show in the natural beauty world. It naturally increases the production of collagen within the skin; this helps the skin stay youthful and limits the signs of ageing.

1 tsp avocado oil

Apply instead of your moisturizer to give your skin a revitalizing boost.

Face cream for combination oily skin

The leaves of the aloe vera plant are high in antioxidants such as beta carotene, vitamin C and vitamin E. This helps keep the skin hydrated and improve its natural firmness. Adding any type of citrus essential oil to the blend will give the cream an extra hit of vitamin C, which is so beneficial for your skin's health.

2 tbsp aloe vera gel
2 tbsp whole milk
1 tsp avocado oil
6 drops of grapefruit essential oil
Glass jar

Place the aloe vera gel and milk in a bowl; whisk the ingredients until it forms a creamy consistency. Add the avocado oil and grapefruit essential oil and whisk some more. Place in a glass jar and store in the fridge (can be stored for a week of so). Use as you would your normal moisturizer.

Natural body care

As your skin is your biggest organ, it makes sense to look after it.

Soothing hand salve

Combining natural butters is an excellent way to keep your hands in tip-top condition, especially in the winter

Sam: "I often use this oil before bed; it works its magic throughout the night leaving my skin feeling revitalized."

months. Shea butter especially is like food for the skin: it's full of essential vitamins to stave off premature ageing and it helps the skin heal.

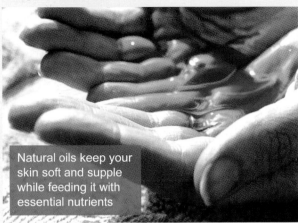

Natural oils keep your skin soft and supple while feeding it with essential nutrients

1 tbsp raw shea butter
1 tbsp raw cocoa butter
1 tbsp beeswax
1 tbsp coconut oil
8 drops of lavender essential oil
Glass jar

In a pan, gently melt the shea butter, cocoa butter, beeswax and coconut oil. Stir all together until everything is completely melted. Add the lavender essential oil. Pour into a clean glass jar. Allow to cool, then use as a normal hand cream or when your hands feel sore. When we think of how often newborn babies like to suck on our fingers, it is worth opting for a non-chemical hand cream when your baby is small.

Vanilla hand scrub

100g (3½oz) brown sugar
60ml (just over 2fl oz) olive oil
1 tsp real vanilla extract
1 tsp vitamin E oil

Mix together the ingredients. Apply the mixture and massage the hands together. This ensures you're removing dead skin from your hands. Massage for around 5 minutes before rinsing well.

Foot soak

Milk makes a really hydrating foot soak. Lactic acid in milk is soothing and nourishing, and as well as being a gentle exfoliator, it softens the feet and removes dead skin. Add some baking soda to enhance the exfoliation effect, leaving your feet feeling amazing.

570ml (20fl oz) whole milk
30g (1oz) baking soda
8 drops of lavender essential oil

Warm the milk in a pan; add the baking soda and essential oil. When warm pour into a bowl big enough for both feet. Test temperature before placing your feet in the bowl. Sit back and relax.

Foot scrub

This scrub will really put the spring back in your step! It will leave your feet feeling soft and fresh.

200g (7oz) brown sugar
115ml (4fl oz) olive oil
10 drops of peppermint essential oil

Mix together the ingredients. Apply the mixture to your feet; massage well for around 5 minutes per foot. Rinse off and moisturize.

Lip care

1 tbsp shea butter
2 tbsp coconut oil

1 tbsp beeswax
1 tsp vitamin E oil
5 drops of grapefruit essential oil

In a pan, gently heat the shea butter and coconut oil. Once melted add the beeswax, and stir continuously until the beeswax has melted. Add the vitamin E and essential oil. Remove from the heat, pour into a container of your choice and let cool. Use when needed.

Body butter

As you can probably tell, we are massive fans of coconut oil. It has so many health benefits, it's great to cook with but also incredible for your skin. Here's a lovely body butter that will leave your skin feeling baby-soft.

2 tbsp cocoa butter
2 tbsp coconut oil

In a pan gently melt the cocoa butter, then remove from heat. Add the coconut oil and stir well, allowing the coconut oil to melt into the mixture. Allow to cool in the fridge for around 20 minutes. Once cooled, whisk the ingredients until it whips into a lovely fluffy butter (a fork will work eventually if you don't have an electric whisk). Spoon into a container of your choice and use when required.

Good morning body scrub

This scrub is ideal to use in the shower, especially in the morning. Lemon is great for waking you up. It works as a natural disinfectant and the scrub will cleanse clogged pores, leaving you ready for your day ahead.

200g (7oz) brown sugar
100g (3½oz) sea salt
2 tbsp lemon juice
2 tbsp coconut oil

Mix the ingredients together into a paste. Apply on damp skin, scrubbing in circular motions and rinse with warm water.

Warning: Only use on your body, sea salt is not recommended for your face.

Rejuvenating honey bath milk

The lactic acid found naturally in milk is soothing and nourishing and a gentle exfoliator for the skin.

350ml (12½fl oz) whole milk
2 tbsp baking soda (soothes and softens the skin)
2 tbsp sea salt
2 tbsp warm honey (anti-inflammatory)

Whisk together and use immediately: pour all ingredients under warm running bath water. Relax and see your skin come to life.

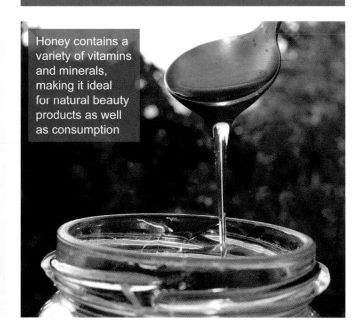

Honey contains a variety of vitamins and minerals, making it ideal for natural beauty products as well as consumption

Final thoughts

In many ways, writing this book has been a lot like having a baby: sharing a dream and devoting our time together to make it happen. The path to finishing a book can be riddled with self-doubt, just like becoming a parent! It helped to have someone else to share the adventure with who was rooting for us all the way.

We hope that you have enjoyed reading this book as much as we have loved writing it. We hope that you feel more ready to take on the most incredible journey of your life. Don't ever lose faith in who you are as a parent and remember that it's a learning curve for all of us. Armed with your love and your determination to do what's best for your children, you have everything that you need.

We'll be continuing on our quest to empower women and their birth partners and to help you through each stage of your baby's development (see our website for further resources). In the meantime, we wish you all the luck in the world.

Holly & Sam xxx

www.naturalmumma.com

Acknowledegments

Sam: "I would like to thank so many special people in my life who have made important contributions to this book, especially my three children Ella, Yasmin and Max. I love you all to the moon and back. To my good friend Holly, who worked tirelessly by my side editing, researching and creating this book, I'm so grateful to have met such a wonderful person and been given the opportunity to work with a talented writer. To my husband Sam, for all the support he gives me with my work. To my parents, who gave me more than I realized – thank you for all your support throughout my life. To my mother-in-law June, thank you for all your support and kindness. To my gran, who is no longer with us (but I miss her every day): you would have been so proud of me; you always told me I could do anything. I just wish you were here to share it with me. To my good friend Vikki, thank you for all your support, guidance and positivity. You keep me grounded and focused.

And thank you to the wonderful team at Green Books, particularly Niall Mansfield, Lindsey Tate, Sheila Stickley, Ada Coghen and Sadie Mayne."

Holly: "Endless love and gratitude to my daughter Jasmine. Being your mum is the best thing that I have ever done. Your creativity and beauty make me eternally proud. Deepest love to Adam, my husband. Thank you always for your perpetual patience and for constantly believing in me. So much love and gratitude to my beautiful friend and co-author Sam. You are an inspiration and it has been a joy working with you on this project. I can't wait to embark on future adventures with you. So much love to my darling parents, Heather and Paul, for raising me in a house that was full of love and books, for caring about the wider world and for showing endless compassion. Your strength has always inspired me. Much love to my treasured in-laws, Paul, Tess and Rhiannon, for being so full of life and love and welcoming me and Jazz into your beautiful family with open arms. Eternal love to my brother, Joe, for making me believe in something bigger and for sparking my creative spirit. I've come a long way since we used to make hand-drawn books at home. I know you'd be proud of who I've become. So much gratitude to Steve for having absolute faith in me and gently suggesting that I become a writer. Your support, guidance and advice have been invaluable. So much love and many thank yous to our glorious models: you were all delightful and made this book a real pleasure to work on.

A special mention to Marilyn, who introduced me to the idea of active birth and whose wisdom and passion led to such an ecstatic first birth experience. Also, to Melinda, whose grounded and balanced approach to complementary therapies was a real source of inspiration. You taught me so much and I will always be grateful for it. A massive shout out to everyone who has encouraged, inspired or supported me over the years. Lastly, thank you to everyone at Green Books for their devotion to our project. It's been an absolute pleasure."

Resources

Complementary therapies

1 Tiffany Field, "Pregnancy and labor massage," *Expert Review of Obstetrics & Gynecology* 5, no. 2 (March 2010): 177-181, doi: 10.1586/eog.10.12

2 NHS Choices, "NICE recommends home births for some mums," (December 2014), http://www.nhs.uknews/2014/12December/Pages/NICE-recommend-homes-births-for-some-mums.aspx

3 Geradine Simkins, "New studies confirm safety of home birth with midwives in the U.S.," Midwives Alliance North America (January 2014), http://mana.org/blog/home-birth-safety-outcomes

4 Marian F MacDorman et al., "Trends in out-of-hospital births in the United States, 1990-2012," National Center for Health Statistics, NCHS Data Brief 144 (March 2014), http://www.cdc.gov/nchs/products/databriefs/db144.htm

5 Homebirth: *Globe and Mail*, "a labour of love few Canadian parents are pursuing," (December 2013), http://www.theglobeandmail.com/life/parenting/home-birth-a-labour-of-love-few-canadian-parents-are-taking/article16050641/

6 Babycenter, "Can anyone have a homebirth?" (April 2015), http://www.babycenter.com.au/a536331/homebirth#ixzz46vto16Q6

7 Ministry of Health, "Report on maternity, 2010," (November 2012), http://www.health.govt.nz/publication/report-maternity-2010

8 Kate Fox, "The smell report," Social Issues Research Centre, http://www.sirc.org/publik/smell_emotion.html

9 Allison England, "Advice and cautions on essential oils," Allison England Aromatherapy, http://vista-1583686.innuity.com/page/1m1io/Essential_oil_info/Advice.html

10 Massagetherapy.com, "Benefits of massage," originally published in *Body Sense* (2001), http://www.massagetherapy.com/articles/index.php?article_id=468

11 Jenifer Worden, "Pregnancy and labour, it's baby time," British Homeopathic Association, http://www.britishhomeopathic.org/bha-charity/how-we-can-help/articles/pregnancy-and-labour/

12 University of Portsmouth, "Reflexology reduces feelings of pain," (April 2013), http://uopnews.port.ac.uk/2013/04/09/reflexology-reduces-feelings-of-pain/

13 Glenys Underwood, "Case-study: reflexology to help sub-fertility," Positive Health Online (February 2009), http://www.positivehealth.com/article/case-studies/case-study-reflexology-to-help-sub-fertility

14 Natural Pregnancy Midwife, "Ways to induce labor naturally," (2016), http://www.natural-pregnancy-midwife.com/ways-to-induce-labor.html

15 M Dolatian et al., "The effect of reflexology on pain intensity and duration of labor on primiparas," *Iranian Red Crescent Medical Journal* 13, no. 7 (July 2011): 475-479, http://www.ncbi.nlm.nih.gov/pmc/articles/PMC3371987/

16 Dr. Mike Berkley, "Infertility and acupuncture," American Pregnancy Association (2015), http://americanpregnancy.org/infertility/acupuncture/

17 Skin Deep Cosmetics Database, "Sodium laureth sulfate," EWG, http://www.ewg.org/skindeep/ingredient.php?ingred06=706089

18 Karen Eisenbraun, "Dangers of sodium lauryl sulfate," Livestrong.com (January 2015), http://www.livestrong.com/article/174367-dangers-of-sodium-lauryl-sulfate/

19 P D Darbre et al., "Concentrations of parabens in human breast tumours," Journal of Applied Toxicology 24, no. 1 (Jan–Feb 2004): 5-13, http://www.ncbi.nlm.nih.gov/pubmed/14745841

20 Farhaan Hafeeze and Howard Maibach, "An overview of parabens and allergic contact dermatitis," Skin Therapy Letter 18, no. 5 (2013), http://www.skintherapyletter.com/2013/18.5/2.html

21 Rachel Nall, "Topical retinol and pregnancy," Livestrong.com (June 2015), http://www.livestrong.com/article/460397-topical-retinol-pregnancy/

22 Medicines and Healthcare Products Regulatory Agency, Gov.uk, "Oral retinoids: pregnancy prevention – reminder of measures to minimise teratogenic risk," (June 2013), http://www.gov.uk/drug-safety-update/oral-retinoids-pregnancy-prevention-reminder-of-measures-to-minimise-teratogenic-risk

23 Charlotte Vøhtz, "Essential guide to ingredients to avoid in baby products," Green People.co.uk, http://www.greenpeople.co.uk/beauty-hub/blog/essential-guide-to-ingredients-to-avoid-in-baby-products

24 Linda F Palmer, "Bonding matters ... the chemistry of attachment," Babyreference.com (August 2013), http://babyreference.com/bonding-matters-the-chemistry-of-attachment/

Preparing for pregnancy

1 NCT, "Hormones in labour," http://www.nct.org.uk/birth/hormones-labour

2 Clare Wilson, "Even low levels of stress could cause infertility," *New Scientist* (March 2014), http://www.newscientist.com/article/dn25274-even-low-levels-of-stress-could-cause-infertility/

3 N J Sebire et al., "Maternal obesity and pregnancy outcome," *International Journal of Obesity* 25, no. 8 (August 2001): 1175-1182, http://www.nature.com/ijo/journal/v25/n8/full/0801670a.html

4 NHS Choices, "New weight advice for pregnancy," (July 2010), http://www. nhs.uk/news/2010/July07/ Pages/new-nice-guidelines-weight-pregnancy.aspx

5 London School of Hygiene & Tropical Medicine, "Mother's diet modifies her child's DNA," (April 2014), http:// www.lshtm.ac.uk/newsevents/ news/2014/mothers_diet.html

6 *Pediatrics*, "Folic acid for the prevention of neural tube defects," 104, no. 2 (1999), http://pediatrics.aappublications. org/content/104/2/325

7 National Institute on Alcohol Abuse and Alcoholism, "Alcohol's effects on the body," http:// www.niaaa.nih.gov/alcohol-health/alcohols-effects-body

8 Department of Health, "Updated alcohol consumption guidelines give new advice on limits for men and pregnant women," (January 2016), https:// www.gov.uk/government/news/ new-alcohol-guidelines-show-increased-risk-of-cancer

9 University of California San Francisco Medical Center, "Substance use during pregnancy," https:// www.ucsfhealth.org/ education/substance_use_ during_pregnancy/

10 Joseph G Allen et al., "Flavoring chemicals in e-cigarettes: diacetyl, 2,3-pentanedione, and acetoin in a sample of 51

products, including fruit-, candy-, and cocktail-flavored e-cigarettes," *Environmental Health Perspectives*, http:// ehp.niehs.nih.gov/15-10185/

11 NHS Direct Wales, "Smoking (quitting)," (October 2015), http://www.nhsdirect.wales. nhs.uk/encyclopaedia/s/ article/smoking(quitting)/

12 Cancer Research UK, "Smoking facts and evidence," (March 2015), http://www. cancerresearchuk.org/ about-cancer/causes-of-cancer/smoking-and-cancer/smoking-facts-and-evidence#smoking_facts6

13 Adrian Burton, "Does the smoke ever really clear? Third-hand smoke exposure raises new concerns," *Environmental Health Perspectives* 119, no. 2 (February 2011), doi: 10.1289/ehp.119-a70

14 British Pregnancy Advisory Service, "Your fertility questions answered," https://www. bpas.org/more-services-information/fertility-qa/

15 Peter Saltta et al., "Is there a true concern regarding the use of hair dye and malignancy development?" *Journal of Clinical and Aesthetic Dermatology* 6, no. 1 (January 2013), http:// www.ncbi.nlm.nih.gov/pmc/ articles/PMC3543291/

Self-care

1 American Society of Anesthesiologists, "Most healthy

women would benefit from light meal during labor," (2015), https://www.asahq.org/ about-asa/newsroom/news-releases/2015/10/eating-a-light-meal-during-labor

2 Lucy Ward, "Mother's stress harms foetus, research shows," *Guardian* (31 May 2007), https://www.theguardian. com/science/2007/ may/31/childrensservices. medicineandhealth

3 Paul Grossman et al., "Mindfulness-based stress reduction and health benefits. A meta-analysis," *Journal of Psychosomatic Research* 57 (2004): 35-43, http://www. academia.edu/1492263/ Mindfulness-based_stress_ reduction_and_health_ benefits._A_meta-analysis._ Grossman_P._Niemann_L._ Schmidt_S._Walach_H._2004_ Journal_of_Psychosomatic_ Research_57_35-43

4 Adrienne A Taren et al., "Dispositional mindfulness co-varies with smaller amygdala and caudate volumes in community adults," *Plos One* 8, no. 5 (22 May 2013), http://dx.doi.org/10.1371/ journal.pone.0064574

5 Daniel J Siegel, "Mindfulness training and neural integration: differentiation of distinct streams of awareness and the cultivation of well-being," *Social Cognitive and Affective Neuroscience* 2, no. 4 (2007): 259-263, http://scan.oxfordjournals. org/content/2/4/259.full

The first trimester

1 George Krucik, ed., "What bodily changes can you expect during pregnancy?" Healthline (4 June 2012), http://www. healthline.com/health/pregnancy/ bodily-changes-during# CirculatorySystemChanges4

2 Frank C Greiss, "Uterine and placental blood flow," Global Library of Women's Medicine (2008), http://www. glowm.com/section_view/ heading/Uterine%20 and%20Placental%20 Blood%20Flow/item/197

3 Baby Center, "Dizziness and fainting during pregnancy," (November 2015), http:// www.babycenter.com/0_ dizziness-and-fainting-during-pregnancy_228.bc

4 Krucik, "Bodily changes during pregnancy."

5 Baby Center, "Frequent urination during pregnancy," (November 2015), http:// www.babycenter.com/0_ frequent-urination-during-pregnancy_237.bc

6 Baby Center, "Breathlessness in pregnancy," (July 2014), http:// www.babycenter.com.au/a219/ breathlessness-in-pregnancy

7 What to Expect, "Stuffy nose and nosebleeds during pregnancy," (2014), http://www. whattoexpect.com/pregnancy/ symptoms-and-solutions/ nasal-congestion.aspx

8 Wikihow, "How to stop nausea with acupressure," http://www.wikihow.com/Stop-Nausea-With-Acupressure

9 Baby Centre, "Sinusitis (natural remedies)," (2015), http://www.babycentre.co.uk/a549318/sinusitis-natural-remedies

10 Cheryl Macdonald, "Why yoga makes mummies happy," http://www.yogabellies.co.uk/?s=why+yoga+makes+mums+happy

11 U.S. Food and Drug Administration, "What you need to know about mercury in fish and shellfish," (March 2004), http://www.fda.gov/food/resourcesforyou/consumers/ucm110591.htm

12 NHS Choices, "Why do I need folic acid in pregnancy?" (March 2015), http://www.nhs.uk/chq/Pages/913.aspx?CategoryID=54&SubCategoryID=129

13 United Healthcare, "Folic acid, calcium and iron," (2016), http://www.healthy-pregnancy.com/uhc/pregnancy/245.shtml

14 Xiaoping Weng et al., "Maternal caffeine consumption during pregnancy and the risk of miscarriage: a prospective cohort study," *American Journal of Obstetrics & Gynecology* 198, no. 3 (March 2008), http://dx.doi.org/10.1016/j.ajog.2007.10.803

15 Mayo Clinic, "Caffeine content for coffee, tea, soda and more," http://www.mayoclinic.org/healthy-lifestyle/nutrition-and-healthy-eating/in-depth/caffeine/art-20049372

16 Kevin Gianni, "7 toxic food additives to avoid," Renegade Health (July 2012), http://renegadehealth.com/blog/2012/07/23/7-toxic-food-additives-to-avoid

17 NHS, "Eat less saturated fat," (June 2015), http://www.nhs.uk/Livewell/Goodfood/Pages/Eat-less-saturated-fat.aspx

18 Dr. Axe, "10 proven manuka honey uses and benefits," Dr. Axe.com, http://draxe.com/manuka-honey-benefits-uses/

19 Medic 8, "Pregnancy calendar," http://www.medic8.com/healthguide/pregnancy-birth/pregnancy/calendar.html

The second trimester

1 Kristeen Cherney, "The second trimester: constipation, gas, and heartburn," http://www.healthline.com/health/pregnancy/second-trimester-constipation-gas-heartburn

2 Kidspot, "Early pregnancy symptom: blood flow," http://www.kidspot.com.au/birth/pregnancy/signs-and-symptoms/early-pregnancy-symptom-blood-flow

3 Dr. Mercola, "How essential oils can improve your life," Mercola.com (August 2015), http://articles.mercola.com/sites/articles/archive/2015/08/17/essential-oils-improve-life.aspx

4 NHS Choices, "Indigestion and heartburn in pregnancy," (November 2014), http://www.nhs.uk/conditions/pregnancy-and-baby/pages/indigestion-heartburn-pregnant.aspx

5 Home Remedies for Life, "Oatmeal for acid reflux," (January 2016), http://homeremediesforlife.com/oatmeal-for-acid-reflux/

6 Dr Colin Tidy, "Anaemia," Patient (2013), http://patient.info/health/anaemia-leaflet

7 Amber Tresca, "Benefits to sleeping on the left side," Love to Know (2016), http://sleep.lovetoknow.com/Sleep_on_the_Left_Side

8 Medic 8, "Pregnancy calendar," http://www.medic8.com/healthguide/pregnancy-birth/pregnancy/calendar.html

The third trimester

1 NHS Choices, "Pre-eclampsia," (2015), http://www.nhs.uk/conditions/Pre-eclampsia/pages/introduction.aspx

2 NCT "Bleeding after birth guide: what to expect," https://www.nct.org.uk/parenting/guide-blood-loss-after-birth

3 Jaclyn M Coletta et al., "Omega-3 fatty acids and pregnancy," *Obstetrics & Gynecology* 3, no. 4 (2010): 163–71, http://www.ncbi.nlm.nih.gov/pmc/articles/PMC3046737/

4 Dr. Mercola, "Pregnant women aren't getting enough omega-3," Mercola.com (April 2015), http://articles.mercola.com/sites/articles/archive/2015/04/27/omega-3-pregnant-women.aspx

5 M Parsons et al., "Raspberry leaf and its effect on labour: safety and efficacy," *Australian College of Midwives Incorporated Journal* 12, no. 3 (September 1999), http://www.ncbi.nlm.nih.gov/pubmed/10754818

6 Baby Centre, "Can raspberry leaf tea bring on labour?" http://www.babycentre.co.uk/x1048118/can-raspberry-leaf-bring-on-labour#ixzz3zfjujRxH

7 Josie L Tenor, "Methods for cervical ripening and induction of labor," *American Family Physician* 67, no. 10 (May 2003): 2123-2128, http://www.aafp.org/afp/2003/0515/p2123.html

8 American Pregnancy Association, "Pregnancy week 30," http://americanpregnancy.org/week-by-week/30-weeks-pregnant/

9 Amy Fleming, "How a child's food preferences begin in the womb," *Guardian* (April 2014), http://www.theguardian.com/lifeandstyle/wordofmouth/2014/apr/08/child-food-preferences-womb-pregnancy-foetus-taste-flavours

10 Michelle Roberts, "Babies can hear syllables in the womb," BBC News (February 2013), http://www.bbc.co.uk/news/health-21572520

11 American Pregnancy Association, "Fetal development: third trimester," http://americanpregnancy.org/while-pregnant/third-trimester/

Your active birth

1 NHS Choices, "Signs that labour has begun," (January 2015), http://www.nhs.uk/conditions/pregnancy-and-baby/pages/labour-signs-what-happens.aspx

2 What to Expect, "Childbirth stage 1: the phases of labor," (2015), http://www.whattoexpect.com/pregnancy/labor-and-delivery/childbirth-stages/three-phases-of-labor.aspx

3 Emma Dufficy, "Should I have a managed or physiological third stage?" Baby Centre (October 2011), http://www.babycentre.co.uk/x562146/should-i-have-a-managed-or-physiological-third-stage

4 NCT, "Pain relief in labour," https://www.nct.org.uk/birth/pain-relief-during-labour

5 Baby Centre, "Entonox (gas and air)," (March 2016), http://www.babycentre.co.uk/a542569/entonox-gas-and-air#ixzz45momMKeF

6 Sam McCulloch, "Using gas during labour – pros and cons," Belly Belly, http://www.bellybelly.com.au/birth/using-gas-during-labour/

7 B Jacobson et al., "Opiate addiction in adult offspring through possible imprinting after obstetric treatment," British Medical Journal 301, no. 6760 (November 1990): 1067-1070, http://www.ncbi.nlm.nih.gov/pmc/articles/PMC1664218/

8 Baby Centre, "Pethidine," (March 2016), http://www.babycentre.co.uk/a542577/pethidine#ixzz45n3HhrEd

9 Baby Centre, "Mobile epidural," (March 2016), http://www.babycentre.co.uk/a542575/mobile-epidural#ixzz45mvYjUgt

10 Michelle J K Osterman and Joyce A Martin, "Epidural and spinal anesthesia use during labor: 27-state reporting area," National Vital Statistics Reports 59, no. 5 (April 2011), http://www.cdc.gov/nchs/data/nvsr/nvsr59/nvsr59_05.pdf

11 Marcos Silva and Stephen H Halpern, "Epidural analgesia for labor: current techniques," Local and Regional Anesthesia 3 (December 2010): 143-153, doi: 10.2147/LRA.S10237

12 Oh Baby! "Epidural," http://www.ohbaby.co.nz/pregnancy/labour-and-birth/pain-relief-in-labour/epidural/

13 Kim Lock, "Caesarean rates are too high. We should not treat birth as a medical procedure," Guardian (22 May 2015), http://www.theguardian.com/commentisfree/2015/may/22/caesarean-rates-are-too-high-we-should-not-treat-birth-as-a-medical-procedure

14 Baby Centre, "Mobile epidural."

15 NHS Choices, "Pain relief in labour," (January 2015), http://www.nhs.uk/conditions/pregnancy-and-baby/pages/pain-relief-labour.aspx

16 Baby Centre, "Spinal," (March 2016), http://www.babycentre.co.uk/a542579/spinal

17 V A Rahm et al., "Plasma oxytocin levels in women during labor with or without epidural analgesia: a prospective study," Acta Obstetricia et Gynecologica Scandinavica 81, no. 11 (November 2002): 1033-1039, http://www.ncbi.nlm.nih.gov/pubmed/12421171

18 Baby Centre, "Epidural," (February 2016), http://www.babycentre.co.uk/a542571/epidural

19 D J Baumgarder et al., "Effect of labor epidural anesthesia on breastfeeding of healthy full-term newborns delivered vaginally," Journal of the American Board of Family Practice 16, no. 1 (Jan–Feb 2003): 7-13, http://www.ncbi.nlm.nih.gov/pubmed/12583645

20 Institute for Quality and Efficiency in Healthcare, "Pregnancy and birth: epidurals and painkillers for labor pain relief," (July 2012), http://www.ncbi.nlm.nih.gov/pubmedhealth/PMH0072751/

21 Denis Campbell, "It's good for women to suffer the pain of a natural birth, says medical chief," Observer (12 July 2009)

22 Unicef global databases (2015), http://www.data.unicef.org/nutrition/iycf.html

23 Unicef, "Breastfeeding," (July 2015), http://www.unicef.org/nutrition/index_24824.html

24 WHO, "Optimal timing of cord clamping for the prevention of iron deficiency anaemia in infants," http://www.who.int/elena/titles/full_recommendations/cord_clamping/en/

25 Y Wang and S Zhao, Vascular Biology of the Placenta, Morgan & Claypool Life Sciences (2010), http://www.ncbi.nlm.nih.gov/books/NBK53250/

26 Mark Sloan, "Common objections to delayed cord clamping – what's the evidence say?" Science and Sensibility (April 2016), https://www.scienceandsensibility.org/p/bl/et/blogid=2&blogaid=526

27 R Grajeda et al., "Delayed clamping of the umbilical cord improves hematologic status of Guatemalan infants at 2 months of age," American Journal of Clinical Nutrition 65, no. 2 (February 1997): 425-431, http://www.ncbi.nlm.nih.gov/pubmed/9022526

28 WHO, "WHO statement on caesarean section rates," (April 2015), http://www.who.int/reproductivehealth/publications/maternal_perinatal_health/cs-statement/en/

29 WHO, "WHO statement on caesarean section rates: frequently asked questions" (April 2015), http://www.who.int/reproductivehealth/topics/maternal_perinatal/faq-cs-section/en/

30 Midwives Alliance of North America, "Legal status of US midwives," http://mana.org/about-midwives/legal-status-of-us-midwives

31 Baby Center, "Home birth and midwifery," (March 2010), http://www.babycenter.ca/a536331/home-birth-and-midwifery#ixzz48FBv7YQ5

32 New Zealand College of Midwives, "About Lead Maternity Carer (LMC) services," (2016), https://www.midwife.org.nz/women-in-new-zealand/about-lead-maternity-carer-lmc-services

33 Jane Palmer, "Australian homebirth is in danger," Pregnancy, Birth and Beyond, http://www.pregnancy.com.au/midwifery/musings-of-a-midwife/australian-homebirth-is-in-danger.shtml

Your new arrival

1 Baby Centre, "Bonding after birth," (August 2014), http://www.babycentre.co.uk/a658/bonding-after-birth

2 Marcelle Pick, "Postpartum depression," WomentoWomen.com, https://wwwwomentowomen.com/emotions-anxiety-mood/postpartum-depression/

3 Miranda Hitti, "Baby's nose knows mom's smell," Web MD (2005), http://www.webmd.com/parenting/baby/news/20050706/babys-nose-knows-moms-smell

4 Heather Hitchcock, "Colostrum and the stages of breast milk," Livestrong.com (October 2013), http://www.livestrong.com/article/496122-colostrum-and-the-stages-of-breast-feeding/

5 Unicef, "Benefits of skin-to-skin contact for preterm babies," http://www.unicef.org.uk/BabyFriendly/Health-Professionals/going-baby-friendly/FAQs/Breastfeeding-FAQ/Benefits-of-skin-to-skin-contact-for-preterm-babies-/

6 Stephanie Watson, "Caring for your child's eczema," Web MD (2014), http://www.webmd.com/skin-problems-and-treatments/eczema/child-eczema-14/baby-diet

7 NHS, "Cradle cap," (March 2015), http://www.nhs.uk/conditions/cradle-cap/Pages/Introduction.aspx

8 RecyclingBins.co.uk, "Recycling facts," http://www.recyclingbins.co.uk/recycling-facts/

9 Baby Centre, "Which sunscreens are best for my baby?" (April 2014), http://www.babycentre.co.uk/x561727/which-sunscreens-are-best-for-my-baby

The babymoon

1 Yeoun Soo Kim-Godwin, "Postpartum beliefs and practices among non-Western cultures," Birthways (2003), http://www.birthways.com/girlnet_docs/Postpartum_Beliefs.pdf

2 Attachment Parenting International, "What is attachment parenting?" (2013), http://www.attachmentparenting.org/WhatIsAP.php

3 Attachment Parenting International, "Prepare for pregnancy, birth, and parenting," (2016), http://www.attachmentparenting.org/principles/principles.php

4 Rosie Knowles, "How babywearing can help with postnatal depression," Sheffield Sling Surgery (March 2015), http://www.sheffieldslingsurgery.co.uk/post-natal-depression/

5 U A Hunziker and R G Barr, "Increased carrying reduces infant crying: a randomized controlled trial," Pediatrics 77, no. 5 (May 1986), http://pediatrics.aappublications.org/content/77/5/641

6 Ask Dr. Sears, "Benefits of babywearing," http://www.askdrsears.com/topics/health-concerns/fussy-baby/baby-wearing/benefits-babywearing

7 Guinevere Webster, "All about babywearing," Oxford Sling Library (2008), http://www.oxfordslinglibrary.co.uk/all-about-babywearing/

8 Chris Molnar, "Kangaroo care and premature babies," Parenting Journals (July 2007), http://www.parenting-journals.com/26/kangaroo-care-and-premature-babies/

9 Ask Dr. Sears, "Benefits of babywearing."

10 NICE, "Empowering families to make informed choices on co-sleeping with babies," (December 2014), https://www.nice.org.uk/news/press-and-media/empowering-families-informed-choices-co-sleeping-babies

11 NCT, "Co-sleeping safety," https://www.nct.org.uk/parenting/co-sleeping-safely-your-baby

12 Australian Breastfeeding Association, "Breastfeeding, co-sleeping and sudden unexpected deaths in infancy," (2013), https://www.breastfeeding.asn.au/bfinfo/breastfeeding-co-sleeping-and-sudden-unexpected-deaths-infancy

13 NCT, "Co-sleeping safety."

14 Baby Centre, "Co-sleeping and safety," (April 2012), http://www.babycentre.co.uk/a558334/co-sleeping-and-safety

15 Baby Centre, "Co-sleeping and safety."

16 Tiffany Field et al., "Massage therapy for infants of depressed mothers," Infant Behaviour and Development 19, no. 1 (January 1996): 109-114, http://www.blossomandberry.com/benefits/research-supporting-baby-massage/

17 Linda F Palmer, "Bonding matters: the chemistry of attachment," Baby Reference.com (August 2013), http://babyreference.com/bonding-matters-the-chemistry-of-attachment/

18 Baby Centre, "Wind," (2013), http://www.babycentre.co.uk/a567409/wind

Postnatal healing: time for you

1 Lauren Frey Daisley, "Healing hints: what postpartum recovery is really like," (September 2012), http://www.parents.com/pregnancy/my-body/postpartum/healing-after-pregnancy/

2 NCT, "Dads in distress: many new fathers are worried about their mental health," (June 2015), https://www.nct.org.uk/press-release/dads-distress-many-new-fathers-are-worried-about-their-mental-health

Breastfeeding

1 NHS, "Breastfeeding in public," (April 2015), http://www.nhs.uk/conditions/pregnancy-and-baby/pages/breastfeeding-in-public.aspx

2 University of Rochester Medical Center, "Back pain in pregnancy," https://www.urmc.rochester.edu/encyclopedia/content.aspx?ContentTypeID=134&ContentID=52

3 Joseph Pritchard, "Mastitis," Healthline, http://www.healthline.com/health/mastitis#Causes3

4 Melissa Kotlen Nagin, "The content and composition of breast milk," About Health (December 2014), http://breastfeeding.about.com/od/breastfeedingbasics/p/bmcontent.htm

5 NHS Choices, "Tongue-tie," (January 2015), http://www.nhs.uk/Conditions/tongue-tie/Pages/Introduction.aspx

6 Acas, "Accommodating breastfeeding employees in the workplace," (October 2013), http://www.acas.org.uk/media/pdf/2/i/Acas-guide-on-accommodating-breastfeeding-in-the-workplace.pdf

7 Ministry of Health, "Breastfeeding and returning to work," (June 2015), http://www.health.govt.nz/your-health/pregnancy-and-kids/first-year/helpful-advice-during-first-year/breastfeeding-perfect-you-and-your-baby/breastfeeding-and-returning-work

8 Australian Breastfeeding Association, "Can you return to work and still breastfeed?" (July 2013), https://www.breastfeeding.asn.au/bf-info/breastfeeding-and-work/can-you-return-work-and-still-breastfeed

9 INFACT Canada, "Breastfeeding: it's your right!" http://www.infactcanada.ca/breastfeeding_rights.htm

10 NCSL, "Breastfeeding state laws," (December 2015), http://www.ncsl.org/research/health/breastfeeding-state-laws.aspx

Naturally nutritious weaning

1 NHS Choices, "Your baby's first solid foods," (May 2015), http://www.nhs.uk/conditions/pregnancy-and-baby/pages/solid-foods-weaning.aspx

2 NHS Choices, "Your baby's first solid foods."

3 NHS Choices, "Your baby's first solid foods."

4 Wikipedia, "Complete protein," (March 2016), https://en.wikipedia.org/wiki/Complete_protein

5 Vegetarian Society, "Food allergy and intolerance," https://www.vegsoc.org/sslpage.aspx?pid=785

Healing foods: meal plans

1 Kerry Torrens, "The health benefits of nuts," BBC GoodFood.com, http://www.bbcgoodfood.com/howto/guide/health-benefits-nuts

2 Jessie Szalay, "Brown rice: health benefits and nutrition facts," Live Science (April 2015), http://www.livescience.com/50461-brown-rice-health-benefits-nutrition-facts.html

3 Better Health, "Iron deficiency – adults," (September 2014), https://www.betterhealth.vic.gov.au/health/conditionsandtreatments/iron-deficiency-adults

Natural woman: home beauty recipes

1 Home Remedies for Life, "How to remove blackheads quickly with honey," (2015), http://homeremediesforlife.com/honey-for-blackheads/

Further reading

Comfort, Settle and Sleep: The natural way to soothe your baby and care for yourself by Samantha Quinn (Connections, 2014)

Active Birth: The new approach to giving birth naturally by Janet Balaskas (Harvard Common Press, 1994)

Essential Vegan Cookbook by Vanessa Almeida (Neni Design, 2013) http://essentialvegan.uk/

The Food of Love: Your formula for successful breastfeeding by Kate Evans (Myriad Editions, 2008)

Gattefossé's Aromatherapy by René-Maurice Gattefossé, edited by Robert B Tisserand (C W Daniel, 1993)

The No-Nonsense Guide to Green Parenting: How to raise your child, help save the planet and not go mad by Kate Blincoe (Green Books, 2015)

The Green Parent http://thegreenparent.com

Index

Also by Green Books

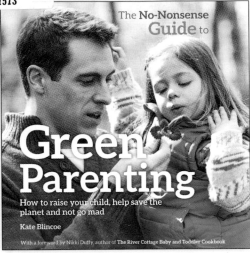

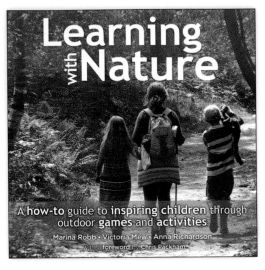

"The ultimate handbook for a fun, green and healthy family."
David Bond, director of The Wild Network

"You will never want to waste a day inside again!"
Jess French, presenter of CBeebies *Mini Beast Adventures*

Ebooks by the same authors

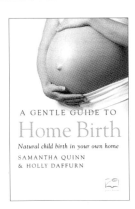

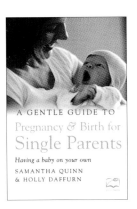

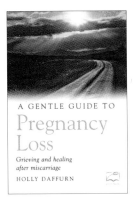

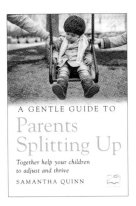

Environmental publishers for over 25 years. For our full range of titles and to order direct from our website, see: *www.greenbooks.co.uk*

Join our mailing list for new titles, special offers, reviews and author events: *www.greenbooks.co.uk/subscribe*

For bulk orders (50+ copies) we offer discount terms. For details, contact: *sales@greenbooks.co.uk*

Send us a book proposal on eco-building, science, gardening, etc.: *www.greenbooks.co.uk/for-authors*

 @Green_Books   /GreenBooks